[Iconographia]

a Franco Maria Ricci edition

HERBARIUM

natural remedies from a medieval manuscript

Texts by
*Adalberto **Pazzini** and **Emma** Pirani*
Original captions by
Ububchasym de Baldach

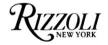
RIZZOLI
NEW YORK

The publisher would like to thank the Biblioteca Casanatense of Rome.

Designed by Franco Maria Ricci
Edited by Laura Casalis
Translated from the Italian by Michael Langley
Colour separation by Zincografia Vaccari, Modena
Text composed in Bodoni Italics
Printed in Milan by GEA S.p.A., February 1980
Published in the United States of America by
RIZZOLI INTERNATIONAL PUBLICATIONS, INC.
712 Fifth Avenue/New York 10019

Library of Congress Catalog Card Number: 79-93004
ISBN: 0-8478-0305-8
Printed in Italy

Introduction

The source of Theatra and Tacuini Sanitatis is to be found in the herbals, bestiaries and lapidaries of the XIVth and XVth centuries, when they were presented as manuscripts which in the course of time were printed and published.

It may seem strange that the word "theatre" should have been used in this context. In common acceptance it denotes an institution with which we are all familiar and which has no connection whatever with medical literature. But in its transferred sense the Latin theatrum means the display or setting out of objects and ideas, of thoughts, feelings and information which are brought to the notice of the public rather as the dramatist airs sentiments and feelings while animating his play with scenic episodes.

Thus Theatrum Sanitatis simply means the exposition of information regarding health to persons moved by curiosity and the desire to study it. The word Tacuinum derives from the Arabic Taqwin, a "tablet" or "list". It offers a summary of useful indications, and this is clearly stated in the original manuscripts.

Here, for example, is a definition of this type of literary-scientific work left us by an early author, Buhahyliha Byngezla of Baghdad, a Christian doctor who died in about 1100. "The Tacuinum is the art of presenting knowledge in a concise and ready form, drawn from experience and related to purposeful ends. It was invented to suit men of our age, especially the rich and noble who ask only for the results of knowledge and are little interested in the probability and theory of a cure. This book is therefore of use to Kings and Magnates in whose rooms it should never fail to find a place."

Another title given to these books was Hortus Sanitatis. This term recalls the old horti simplicium of the monasteries, those gardens of "simples", or medicinal plants, which provided natural remedies for communities whose nursing members cultivated herbs for the cure of their sick brethren. Among the best known of these works is Giovanni da Cuba's Hortus Sanitatis, the first edition of which was published as a herbarium in Mainz in 1484. A better known version, which was shorter, appeared in 1485, also under the title of Hortus Sanitatis. Adorned with charming woodcuts, it won popular favour and was issued in successive editions right up to the end of the XVIIth century. One of the most distinguished works of medical literature of the quattrocento, it propounds the virtues of simples found in the three Kingdoms of Nature, animal, vegetable and mineral.

Nor was there any lack of herbaria of the stamp that aspires to courtly dignity. In their treatment of information a level was attained which, allowing for the wider sense of the word at that time, can be described as "scientific". Works of this kind include De virtutibus herbarum, presented by Macer Floridus as a poem in Latin hexameters, Medicinae libellus by Benedetto Crespo, Archbishop of Milan, and the so-called herbarium of the pseudonymous writer Apuleius. From these and other similar sources fuller herbals were compiled, of which Flos medicinae or Regimen Salernitanum is perhaps the best known.

To give an added attraction to this genre, a supernatural, indeed a magical element was introduced. Herbs, it was said, were subject to astral influences, they had a spiritual, a transcendent life. In the early Middle Ages a magico-medical literature grew up with ancient Alexandria as its inspirational centre. Little by little, descriptions of the medical properties of plants, animals and minerals were amplified to take in the general rules of hygiene regarding food, diet and clothing; advice about the seasons of the year was given; the differing characteristics of men, physiological phenomena and their manifestations were examined; the treatment of certain diseases was discussed; medical notes and other items were inserted by persons interested in padding out the original text.

Of our Theatrum Sanitatis, *which is preserved in the Casanatense Library in Rome, two other copies are known to exist. One belongs to the National Library in Vienna, the other to the Bibliothèque Nationale in Paris, but both bear the title* Tacuinum Sanitatis. *A fourth copy, which has not been traced, may be the one which according to Delisle was once in the Castle Library in Pavia.*

The Casanatense manuscript, which concerns us, bears the imprint "Ms. 4182"; it measures 33x23 cms and consists of 107 pages displaying 208 illustrations. The format is very similar to the Paris version (32.5x25 cms, 103 pages, 208 illustrations) but larger than the Vienna one (24x25 cms, 108 pages, 208 illustrations). However, in its layout and state of preservation the latter approximates more closely to ours. There are also differences in the illustrations: the figures in the Paris manuscript occupy the entire page, while those of the Rome and Vienna versions are framed in red with ample space beneath for descriptive matter.

The author of the text was Ububchasym de Baldach, a corruption of the name Abul Hasan al Muchtar Ibn Botlan, better known in medieval medical literature as Ellucasim Elimittar. Historians who have studied him — among them Choulant, Neuburger and Baglioni — agree that he was a Christian doctor of Baghdad who died either in 1052 or 1063. It is also known that he wrote a treatise similar to the Theatrum *under the title of* Takwin al suha *(or essuha), from which derives the Latin* Tacuinum Sanitatis *or* Tabulae Sanitatis. *It was never published in Arabic. Baldach's manuscript starts with a preface stating the arrangement of the material and the aims of the author: "*Theatrum Sanitatis *concerns the six things necessary to all men for the daily maintenance of health together with rules and ways to attain it." It goes on to say what these six things are: climate... food and drink... activity and rest... sleep and wakefulness... the regulation of the moods of joy and sadness." (Which last might now be called the psychosomatic condition). Illnesses, it is stated, spring from changes in these "six natural things". The author's purpose is to set out briefly and concisely a body of material that has been extracted*

and summarised from the reading of many books: a declaration of intents which is usually found in works of this kind.

There follows an alphabetical index interposed in the manuscript by another much later hand. This gives the main items treated in the text, beginning with a disquisition on medicinal simples and, in particular, on the healing properties of figs and grapes. The first illustration shows the maestro in academic style wearing the costume of his day. Next comes the text proper, or rather the illustrations accompanied by relevant comments and notes. The first ninety-nine of the 208 illustrations contained in the complete Casanatense version are dedicated to simples of the vegetable kingdom. (About fifty of them are published here).

In medical language the term "simple" means any medicament that is not artificially compounded but is administered in its natural state. Even though it may be produced by the hand of man, as wine, cheese, butter and oil are, it is still considered a simple, as distinct from compounds like tetrapharmaco and diatessaron which are composed of four simples, or, again, Apostles' ointment, into which go twelve ingredients, theriaca with ninety-five different substances, and many other preparations.

On reading the descriptions of the plates one may ask what is the meaning of the humour or temperament of a simple. Terms like "cold in the first degree... dry in the second degree... humid in the third degree" are also used. To understand these definitions one should know that temperament was attributed to a medicament no less than to the patient himself. It was determined wholly on observations of the qualities, real or apparent, of the plant. To take rue, the herb of grace, this plant was reputed to have a "hot" humour, but since it contains little moisture it was also described as "dry". The watery lettuce, with its insipid taste, was regarded as having a "cold-moist" humour. According to lexicographers, the word "temperament" corresponds to the Greek crasis, *meaning a combination of humours or, in a broader sense, the constitution of the organism. Its definition as hot, dry, moist or cold comes from the teachings of*

Empedocles, for whom the primary substances were air, earth, fire and water. For greater clarity it was usual to combine two adjectives, the earth being described as "dry-cold", fire as "hot-dry" and water as "moist-cold".

Adhering to a logical process of reasoning, the constitution of the living organism, that is of man and the animals, was endowed with the above properties, and these were attributed to the four humours they were believed to embody, namely: blood, phlegm, yellow bile (choler) and black bile (black choler or melancholy). Blood was considered hot-moist, and phlegm (i.e. catarrh, mucus and anything of a watery nature) was cold-moist. Of a bitter, burning taste, yellow bile was likened to fire and was hot-dry. Melancholy was regarded as the lees or dregs of yellow bile and was described as being cold-dry.

It was on these assumptions that the nature of diseases was defined. They were the result, it was thought, of an imbalance of the humours, or of the deterioration of one of them. Thus fevers were hot-dry, as also was inflammation; cholera nostras (a form of gastro-enteritis) was cold-moist and so on. Cures were based on the application of medicaments of the opposite temperament to the one to be subdued, for which reason the method was known as contraria contrariis. Hence the search among drugs and simples for the right "temperament" to counter a disease and expel it. For example, the hot-dry humour of fever was treated by applying cold-moist poultices of snails to the patient's wrists. As an indication of their efficacy, the "temperament" of these medicaments was classified by degree: first, second and third degree. And it was the Arabs who were the first to grade simples in this way, the object being to apply them according to the gravity of the disease under treatment.

The descriptions that accompany the plates are arranged in such a way as to enable the reader to note the characteristics of each plant and tree in the following order: its nature, temperament and degree; its principal curative qualities; its harmful effects and their remedies.

Adalberto Pazzini

Bibliographical Notes

The Theatrum Sanitatis, which Delisle calls "an illustrated manual of hygiene", is really a glorified Tacuinum, or notebook. In this issue the text has been reduced and the illustrations have been given pride of place. It is intended for a discerning public, for persons who go to it not so much to study these rules of health as to enjoy the aesthetic pleasure that is engendered by a symbolic interpretation.

In this way a charming picture will be formed of daily life in the fields and gardens attached to large houses of the period, in streets and stalls and in the tasks of labourers. How appropriate, then, that the title of Theatrum Sanitatis should always have been used for the illustrated edition of the Tacuinum which is reproduced here. Each chapter, or set of notes, in a book which Toesca called "an illustrated encyclopaedia" gave the old artists their key to depicting characteristic scenes through which, as on a theatre stage, we catch glimpses of the lives of gentlemen, merchants, peasants and gardeners in medieval times.

Only three copies of the illustrated edition of the Tacuinum have come down to us. A comparative examination of their texts and illustrations leaves the impression that they are the product of a well established iconographic tradition. Indeed the surviving copies are probably all that remains of a much larger number commissioned by princely courts, noble families and rich merchants.

The three existing Tacuini are in the National Library, Vienna (New Series 2644), the National Library, Paris (Acq.s Latin 1673) and the Casanatense Library in Rome (mss. 4182). All have been well studied by bibliographers, art critics and *medical historians. The first to do so was Julius Schlosser who, in 1895, published a detailed critique in which he brought the Vienna Tacuinum to the notice of scholars, at the same time attributing the illustrations to Verona art. Delisle's review of this critique, published in the following year in the* Journal des Savants, *was made the occasion by the* Bibliothèque Nationale *to announce its recent acquisition of a* Tacuinum *and to arrange a first comparison between the two copies. Then, in 1908, Antonio Muñoz wrote an article on the Casanatense* Theatrum *in which he discussed its illustrations in the light of the other two. In his opinion Schlosser was correct in attributing them to Veronese artists.*

It is relevant that the stylistic and iconographic similarities of the three manuscripts are so striking that no critic making a close study of one could have avoided referring to the others.

Toesca was the first to refute Schlosser's Verona School theory. He saw in the illustrations the mark of Lombard art and, in particular, of the late 14th-century School of Giovannino de' Grassi, Franco and Filippo de' Veris and Anovelo da Imbonate. With few exceptions. all who have worked on them since Toesca - and they have done so from various standpoints - have accepted this critic's judgement. Moreover, his views have been borne out by other very recent writers, including Mario Salmi and Otto Pächt. For the illustrations in the three Tacuini *clearly demonstrate the characteristics of Lombard art, the more detailed aspects of which were not recognised in Schlosser's day but were gradually confirmed in critical studies made in the years following Toesca's fundamental work. Without examining the illuminator's art too deeply, we would call attention to those common characteristics which are clearly recognisable as being of Lombard origin: the lively and warm-hearted portrayal of landscape and especially of plants and animals; the setting of the figures in realistic surroundings the details of which are themselves realistically shown; the style and fashion of the clothes, the buxom grace and low-cut necklines of the women, the short embroidered tunics and overalls of the men.*

What differences are there between the three works?

The Paris manuscript, which is undoubtedly the richest and most varied, is the work of the best of these artists; from the pictorial and stylistic viewpoints, the other two — the Viennese and Casanatense versions — resemble one another very closely.

The Casanatense illustrations are all of a piece, though they come from different hands, at least three, one of whom can be recognised as the master and two or three as his pupils. Their work, especially the best of it, reveals a painstaking approach to an accurate portrayal of reality. People, plants and animals are set in their surroundings with the utmost naturalness. In general, the balance is correct even if the perspective is often false. The colours are warm and harmonious and the frequent use of white lead in the shadows of the face gives sharpness to the features. A keen sense of nature is ever present, and an almost poetic sense is expressed in the way these artists portray plants and the life of the fields. For example, two similar illustrations depicting wheat (plate XLVI) and barley (plate XLVII) show the changing colours of ripe corn in the breeze, and beneath the ears of the wheat a light sprinkling of colour lent by the flowers. The absence of the human figure from this scene gives it a certain poetic intensity.

In its illustrations the Casanatense Tacuinum *is more faithful to the text than are the others. Pictorially exact, yet true to the iconographic tradition of the period, it steers clear of the frills of fantasy. This is evident if we compare it with the Vienna manuscript, in which the composition of the illustrations is so similar to those of our Casanatense version as to suggest that they are direct derivatives. But that theory can be excluded for reasons which we shall now give. Starting from a reference contained in an inventory of the Visconti Library made in 1426, which mentions a* Tacuinum Sanitatis *since lost, and from an examination of a volume of designs containing figures and scenes that might be the preliminary studies for a* Tacuinum Sanitatis, *(the volume is now in the Accademia Carrara at Bergamo), Mario Salmi suggests that the* Tacuinum *which was once in the Visconti Library was in fact the prototype on which the three existing*

Tacuini were based. This of course is pure conjecture, but it is plausible enough, for the style of Giovannino de' Grassi influenced the illustrative work in the three surviving manuscripts, those of Paris and Vienna in particular, albeit less in the case of the Casanatense exemplar.

While corresponding in general to the iconography of the Vienna illustrations the Casanatense pictures are, as we have said, more consistent in their adherence to the text, more faithful to the reality they represent. Throughout this part of our Theatrum, which is devoted to fruits and herbs, we observe that the trees and plants are shown in isolation without the addition of figures, as in the two other manuscripts. In these the size of the figures is sometimes disproportionate to that of the plants. This is most noticeable in the Paris version where the plants overpower the human figure, so that the basilica and egg plants actually assume the appearance of trees. But then it is in these trees, these plants and fields of grain, standing out in lonely isolation and revealing the loving care with which they were depicted, that the poetry of these illustrations really lies. Men and women seldom intrude, but when they do they are faithfully represented. In our version their movements are never conventional or affected, as in the other two Tacuini. Here they are at complete ease. And that is how it should be. Husbanding their herbs and roots, these country folk fit admirably into scenes in which they play a natural part.

Emma Pirani

Plates

The descriptions accompanying these plates are taken from the Latin captions of Ububchasym de Baldach in the Casanatense manuscript and from notes found in other late medieval herbaria.

I - Ububchasym de Baldach

The Theatre of Health *concerns the six things necessary to all men for the daily maintenance of health together with rules and ways to attain it.*
The first rule is always to breathe good fresh air.
The second is to consume the right food and drink.
The third is regular activity and repose.
The fourth is to refrain from too much sleep and from too much wakefulness.
The fifth concerns the retention and expulsion of the humours.
The sixth is to be moderate in joy, in fear and in anxiety.
The observance of these rules ensures the conservation of good health; their neglect — such is the will of God — leads to sickness and disease.
To these general rules must be added many of a more specific and necessary kind, of which we shall speak, if it please God. We shall speak also of the choices to be made, according to age and constitution.
And here these things will be shown concisely, for the lengthy discourses of learned men often tire the listener, as do the conflicting opinions of many diverse books.
Men want to know only the conclusive results of what concerns them, not demonstrations and definitions. Consequently, it is our intention that this book should contain the essence of longer treatises and summarise the contents of different books. Notwithstanding this, we do not propose to ignore the wise counsels of the ancient physicians.

II - Figs (*Fichus*)

Figs are hot and moist in the first degree.
They are best when of the white variety, the skin of which must be peeled.
They are beneficial in cleansing the kidneys and removing small calculi. A poultice made of dried figs is good for abscesses.
The fig is harmful inasmuch as it creates flatulence and inflates the humours.
Harmful effects are remedied by drinking syrup made with vinegar and brine.

III - Grapes (*Uve*)

Grapes are hot in the first degree, that is moderately so, and moist in the second degree.

The best are those with big pips and fine skins, juicy and unblemished.

They benefit by nourishing and fattening the body while keeping the bowels free.

They do harm by causing thirst and disturbing the bladder and head.

This can be avoided if they are eaten with pomegranates.

IV - Peaches (*Persicha*)

The peach is cold and moist in the second degree.

The best are of the muscatel flavour.

They relieve burning fevers because of their cold-moist nature, and they lubricate the stomach.

Peaches may cause harm by disturbing the humours, but this is overcome by eating them with a little fragrant wine.

V - Pears (*Pira*)

This fruit is cold in the first degree, dry in the second.

The best are "sichaeni" pears, which the Greeks call "sicyoni".

They are good for weak stomachs but harmful to the intestines.

No ill effects ensue if a little garlic is eaten after them.

VI - Pomegranates (*Granata dulcia*)

The pomegranate is by nature cold in the second degree and moist in the first.

The best of all are those that contain most moisture.

Pomegranates are extremely beneficial to an overheated liver.

They are harmful to the chest and voice, though this defect may be obviated by taking "chaloe" with honey.

VII - Quinces (*Citonia*)

The quince is both cold and dry in the second degree.

Fat and fully grown ones are best recommended.

They are beneficial for the cheerfulness they induce and for stimulating the urine.

They check diarrhoea and they promote the menstrual flux.

This fruit may, however, upset the intestines. If so, it should be eaten with sweet dates.

Quinces can be used for making cider.

VIII - Sharp Apples (*Mala acetosa*)

Cold in the second degree and moist in the first, the sharp apple is best when it has a high water content.

Because of their cold-moist nature these apples relieve an overheated liver.

Care should be taken lest they harm the chest and voice.

The remedy is to eat them with "chaloe" sweetened with honey.

IX - Sycamores (*Sicomuri*)

Sycamores, known also as Egyptian figs, yield a medicinal milky white fluid called latex. This fruit is by nature cold and dry in the second degree.

The large dark heads are best and these, in particular, pacify abscesses and boils in the throat. They also mellow the body and relieve snakebite.

But they can provoke stomach pains, with malign effects. This danger is obviated by dosing with "Trifera minore", a mild pain-killer with a bland flavour.

X - Citrons (*Nabach idest cedrum*)

Nabach, as the Arabs call them, are cold and dry in the third degree.

The best citrons, which are chill and dry to the taste, are the large and fragrant ones.

They are useful for quenching a flux of black bile, but are harmful inasmuch as they slow down the digestion.

This is remedied by eating honey fresh from the comb.

XI - Sweet Cherries (*Ceresa dulcia*)

The sweet variety is cold in the first degree and moist at the upper limit of the first, that is, almost in the second degree.

Sweet, ripe cherries are the best.

They are good for the stomach, for they moisten it, are easily digested and soothe the bowels.

But care should be taken not to eat them in excess as their effects may then be unpleasant.

To avert such consequences drink sweet wine with them.

XII - Carob Beans (*Carubee*)

These beans, which are the fruit of the carob or locust tree, are hot in the first degree, dry in the second.

Some people call them St. John's Bread.

The fresh, sweet beans are best.

Beneficial as a laxative when fresh, they have the opposite effect in their dry state.

Carob beans are hard to digest, though this defect can be corrected by eating them with sticks of refined sugar.

XIII - Acorns (*Glandes*)

Acorns are by nature cold in the second degree, dry in the third. Large undamaged ones are recommended.

Imbibed as a decoction they check the flow of dysentery, that is, they assist the power of retention.

Finely pounded for use in vaginal pessaries, they suppress the menstrual flow, which they also do when taken orally.

Acorns do, however, bring on headaches, but this can be overcome by eating them with sugar.

They also provide an effective cure for inflammation if pounded and made into a paste by adding fat.

XIV - Black Olives (*Olive nigre*)

Black olives are moderately hot and tend to dryness. They are best eaten unpickled.

Although they sharpen the appetite they may bring on headaches and sleeplessness, and because they rot quickly they tend to upset the stomach. Eye trouble sometimes follows. All these effects can be avoided by eating them with other dishes.

XV - Chestnuts (*Castanee*)

Chestnuts are hot in the first degree and dry in the second.
The best are the Brianza ones when properly ripe.
Highly nutritious, they stimulate sexual intercourse, but they make the stomach swell and bring on headaches.
If boiled in water, they will have none of these ill effects.

XVI - Pine Cones (*Pinee*)

Hot in the second degree and dry in the first, the best cones have seeds in them.
They alleviate bladder and kidney troubles. They also excite amorous desires.
Worms may be found beneath the outer scales, but not if the tree is properly looked after and pruned.

XVII - Lemons (*Citra*)

Cold in the second degree and dry in the third, lemons are best when they are large and fragrant.
They are good for choleric fluxes, also for noxious fevers when the juice is taken as a syrup.
Distilled lemon water is used for the treatment of the skin, and when imbibed it helps to eliminate intestinal worms.
The juice of unripe lemons breaks up kidney calculi.
The only drawback about this fruit is that it slows down the digestion. It is advisable to take a little honey with them.

XVIII - Dates (*Cefalones idest Datili*)

Dates are cold in the first degree, dry in the second.
The freshest, sweetest fruit is best.
As a decoction, dates of this variety relieve fever and strengthen the patient. They have a soothing effect on the internal organs but are not good for chest or throat.
When eaten in large quantities they provoke headaches, even intoxication. With honey no harmful results ensue.

XIX - Rutab or ripe dates (*Rutab idest Datilus*)

The "rutab" variety is hot in the second degree, moist in the third.
Beneficial in cases of intestinal pain, these dates have little affinity with the blood. A paste made with poppies is the best corrective.

XX - Sweet Melons (*Melones dulces*)

Cold in the second degree and moist in the third, the best come fresh from Samarkand.
Sweet melons break down the calculi that form in the urinary bladder. They also cleanse the skin.
Cut small and mixed with the roots of arum and bryony, to which is added lemon juice and goat's milk, they are used for the distillation of beauty lotions.
The disadvantage of these melons is that they may cause diarrhoea, but this can be checked by drinking a good wine or sharp syrup.

XXI - Pumpkins (*Cucurbitae*)

Both cold and moist in the second degree, pumpkins, which are best when green and fresh, are good thirst quenchers.
When applied to the breasts of women in childbirth they dry up the milk.
Their flowers yield an oil which relieves kidney pains and eases headaches caused by excessive heat.
The burnt residue of dried pumpkins cures genital ulcers, and the juice of fresh ones soothes ear-aches.
They are quick to decompose and to pass through the body.
This can be remedied by eating them with mustard and spices.

XXII - Cabbages (*Caules onati*)

"Caulis", meaning stem, used often to be applied to all cabbage plants.
Of the Brassica genus, cabbages are hot in the first degree, dry in the second.
The best are fresh ones of a greenish yellow colour.
They loosen costive bowels, but any harm they may do to the intestines is prevented by using oil with them.

XXIII - Marrows and Cucumbers (*Cucumeres et citruli*)

Cold and moist in the third degree, the best are the fat and fully grown ones.
They reduce burning fevers and encourage the urinary flow, but they sometimes cause aches and pains in the stomach and intestines.
These effects are not felt if they are eaten with oil and honey.

XXIV - Capers (*Capari*)

Hot in the third degree, dry in the second, capers grow on rough ground and among the ruins of buildings.
They should be picked when fresh and tender. They will then promote urination and, if taken as an infusion, will relieve the pains of sciatica, cramp, rupture and distressing spasms.
As a decoction they ease toothache. Moreover, the juice of the crushed root kills worms when it is instilled into the ears.
Capers may, however, cause injury by drawing blood and sperm into the urine. The antidote for this is to take vinegar.

XXV - Leeks (*Porri*)

Leeks are hot in the third degree and dry in the second. The long and pointed ones are best.
Such benefits as they have are to increase urination and excite the sexual desires.
On the other hand, they dull the brain and the perceptions.
This can be remedied by taking oil of sesame.

XXVI - Onions (*Cepe*)

Hot in the second degree, moist in the third, onions of the white variety are best. They should be succulent and watery.
They have many qualities: their juice, mixed with honey, sharpens the eyesight; inhaled through the nose they clear the head; pounded to a paste with vinegar, rue and honey, they cure dog bites and skin discolouration (vitiligo); and when rubbed on bald patches their juice restores hair growth.
Onions also strengthen the sexual powers.

The only harm they do is to cause headaches, which pass quickly after drinking a little vinegar and milk.

XXVII - Garlic (*Alea*)
Garlic is hot in the second degree and dry in the third.
The best heads are those that have a rather sharp odour.
Use freely in cases of poisoning, but watch for ill effects as garlic expels the humours from the brain and may do so excessively.
The remedy is to take oil and vinegar.

XXVIII - Asparagus (*Sparagus*)
Asparagus is hot and moist in the first degree.
The best stalks are fresh ones with their heads turned slightly earthward.
They have the power of stimulating and improving amorous union and of alleviating constipation.
Asparagus can, however, damage the stomach fibres, to avoid which add suitable seasoning after boiling.

XXIX - Spinach (*Spinachie*)
Cold in the first degree, spinach is best after it has been drenched by rain.
It is good for coughs and chest troubles but may obstruct the digestion.
This can be corrected by frying the leaves lightly and slowly and then seasoning them.

XXX - Beet (*Blete*)
Beet is both hot and dry in the first degree, the best roots being those that are sweet to the taste.
Its juice removes scurf, but it should be eaten in moderation as it dries the blood.
This defect is prevented by using vinegar and mustard.

XXXI - Parsnips (*Pastinace*)
The parsnip is a root that is hot in the second degree and moist in the first.
A winter vegetable, the red sweet parsnip is the best.
While quickening the sexual desires it retards the digestion.
The parsnip should be boiled for a long time to avoid this latter defect.

XXXII - Mushrooms (*Terra tufule*)
Mushrooms are by nature both hot and moist in the third degree.
The best are big ones of the so-called "melongiane" species.
They have the quality of matching all flavours but give rise to disorders caused by black bile.
Cook them with oil, pepper and salt and no ill effects will follow.

XXXIII - Lettuce (*Lactuce*)
The lettuce is cold and moist in the third degree.
The best are those with big greenish-yellow leaves.
Lettuce, which shares some of the qualities of poppies, rectifies sleeplessness and cures gonorrhea. As a drink it relieves the effects of spider and scorpion stings.
If eaten in large quantities lettuce diminishes the power of the sight and of sexual desire.
To neutralise this tendency eat it with celery.

XXXIV - Mustard (*Sinapi*)
Hot and dry in the third degree, the best mustard is of the red variety freshly grown in kitchen gardens.
It is a sure cure for gout in the big toe (podagra), but it harms the brain. To correct this tendency take almonds mixed with vinegar.

XXXV - Galingale (*Galenga*)
Hot in the third degree and dry in the second, this highly aromatic herb has a piquant taste.
Large roots are best and when used as seasoning they benefit sciatica and enhance sexual desire.
Galingale may disturb the heart unless accompanied by greasy foods.

XXXVI - Mint (*Menta*)
Mint is by nature hot and dry in the second degree and best when grown in kitchen gardens.
It fortifies the stomach, inhibits retching, stops the hiccoughs and checks the flow of black bile.
Mixed with polenta, that is maize-meal pudding, it cures abscesses and inflammations of the breast. Used with salt it helps to heal dog bites.
Mint enhances the sexual desires but restricts the seminal vesicles. This drawback can be rectified by eating it with diuretic herbs.

XXXVII - Rue (*Ruta*)
Rue, or herb of grace, is hot and dry in the second degree.
It grows best when planted near to fig trees.
This herb has the merit of sharpening the vision and dispelling flatulence; it eases pains in the body, chest and joints and is effective in cases of poisoning; it soothes inflammation of the vagina and rectum.
But rue can also be harmful. It consumes the sperm and dulls the sexual desires, a drawback to be remedied by taking "simples" known to favour spermatic production.

XXXVIII - Elecampane (*Enula*)
Elecampane of the inula genus is hot and dry in the second degree.
The best part of the plant is the root.
Its merit is that it fortifies the stomach and eases the chest.
Its defect that it can cause headaches.
In case of the latter the antidote is to eat sugared fruits of coriander.

XXXIX - Horehound (*Marubium*)
Hot in the second degree and dry in the third, horehound grows best in open fields.

It is used in the treatment of jaundice; also for coughs of tubercular origin; another benefit is that it improves the eyesight.

Horehound is harmful to the kidneys and bladder, but this can be rectified by using it with cold diuretic preparations.

XL - Absinthe (*Absintium*)

This herb is hot in the first degree and dry in the second.

Absinthe is best when extracted from smooth, white, flat leaves.

It stimulates the appetite and is used to preserve clothes from moths.

The leaves can be eaten alone without ill effects if it is found that the liquid distillate upsets the stomach.

XLI - Sage (*Salvia*)

Hot in the first degree and dry in the second, sage is cultivated in kitchen gardens for its leaves, which are the best part of the plant.

It is considered good for the nerves and in cases of paralysis.

But it is not wholly beneficial as it tends to make the hair fall out.

This undoubted drawback can be avoided by washing the hair with decoctions of myrtle and domestic saffron.

XLII - Violets (*Viole*)

Violets are cold in the first degree, moist in the second.

Deep blue violets thickly surrounded by leaves are regarded as the best.

They do good even to those who merely smell them.

When boiled and drunk as a decoction they help to expel choleric humours.

With illnesses of a catarrhal type they are not advisable, and if ill effects follow these can be remedied by using elder berries.

XLIII - Crocuses (*Crochus*)

Saffron crocuses are hot in the second degree and dry in the first.

They are best when fresh, of subtle smell and good colour, though the colour should have a whitish film to it.

These flowers give solace to the heart, but they tend to stimulate nausea, for the relief of which it is customary to use acetous medicaments.

XLIV - Anise (*Anisum*)

Hot and dry in the third degree, the best anise berries are fresh and fat ones.

The fruit of this herb dispels flatulence, stimulates milky secretions and excites lust.

The drawback is that it causes constipation, though this can be avoided by eating the seeds whole instead of crushing them.

Aniseed relieves ear-aches and headaches. The best qualities come from Crete and Egypt.

XLV - Fennel (*Feniculus*)

Hot and dry in the second degree, fennel is best cultivated in kitchen gardens.

It is good for the sight and for prolonged fevers.

Should it disturb the intestines by causing fluxes, this can be remedied by taking lozenges made of dried locust beans.

Drunk with wine, its juice alleviates snake bite and stimulates menstrual flux.

The seeds of fennel break down bladder stones and check an excessive production of black bile.

XLVI -Wheat (*Furmentum*)

Wheat is hot and moist, both in the second degree.

The large and well-developed grains are the best.

The great value of wheat to mankind goes without saying.

But not everyone knows that it brings abscesses to the head, or that it can be harmful, for it tends to obstruct the fluidity of the humours.

It must be worked thoroughly, then it will harm no one.

XLVII - Barley (*Ordeum*)

Barley is cold and dry, both in the second degree.

Large white grains, freshly gathered, not stored, are best.

Mildly laxative, barley may produce slight pains, but not if it has been roasted.

The flour can be cooked with dried figs in sweetened water to obtain a cure for abscesses.

I

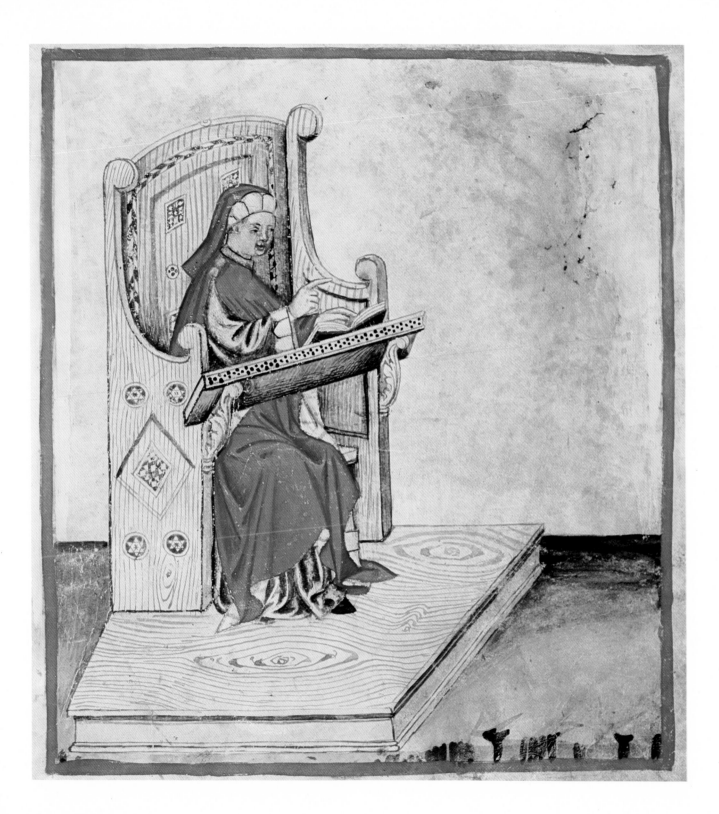

II

Fichus.

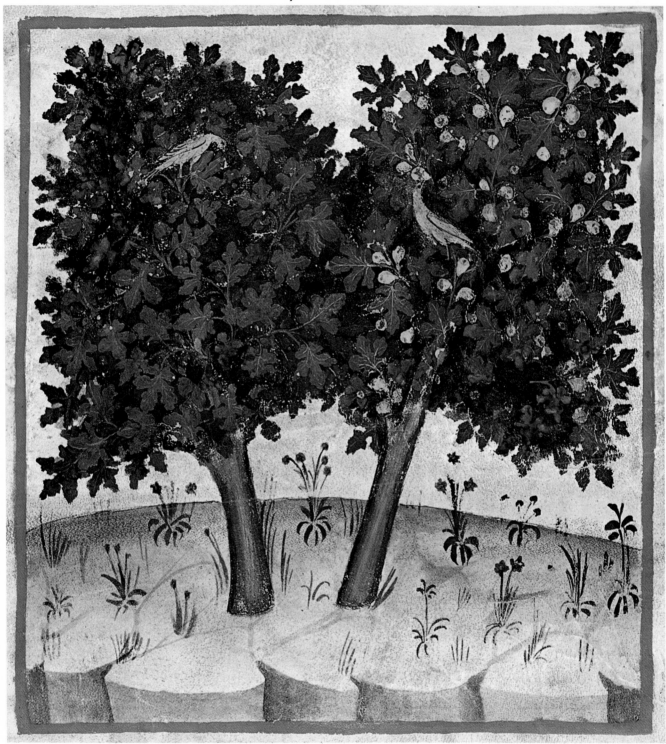

III

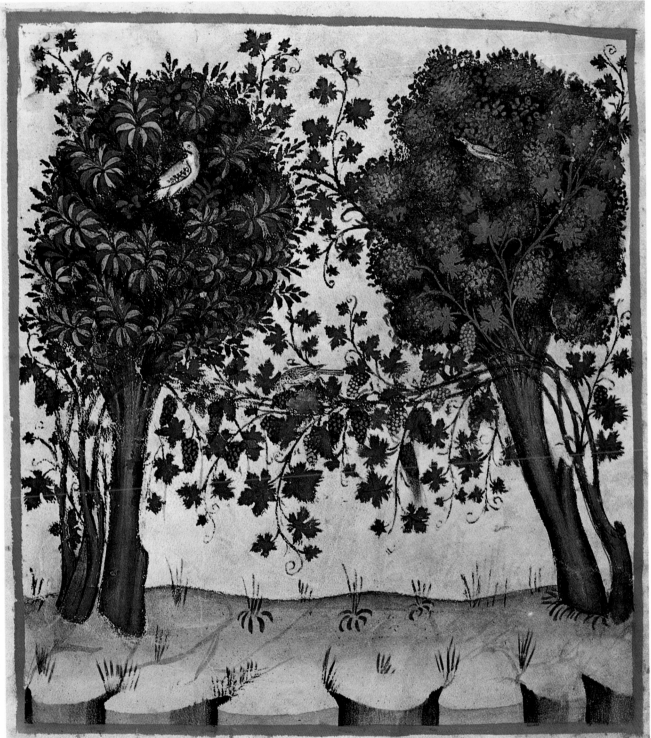

IV

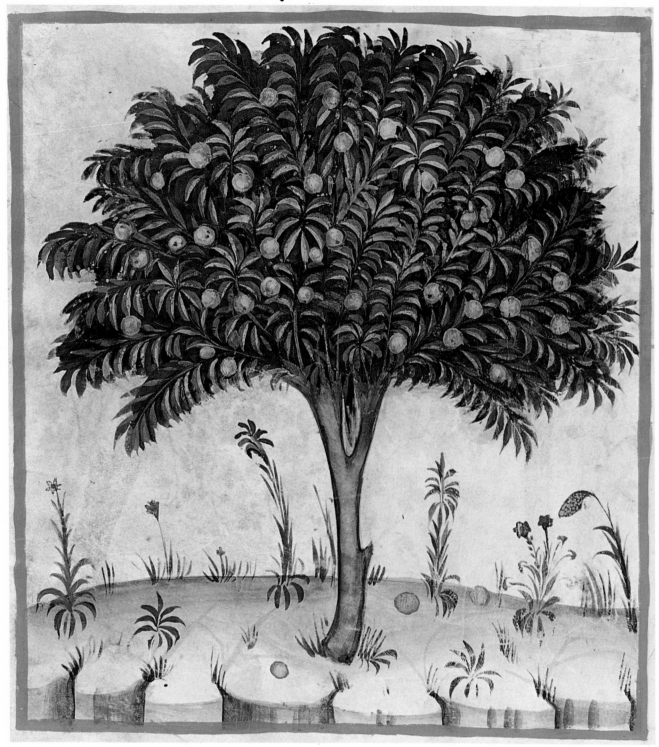

V

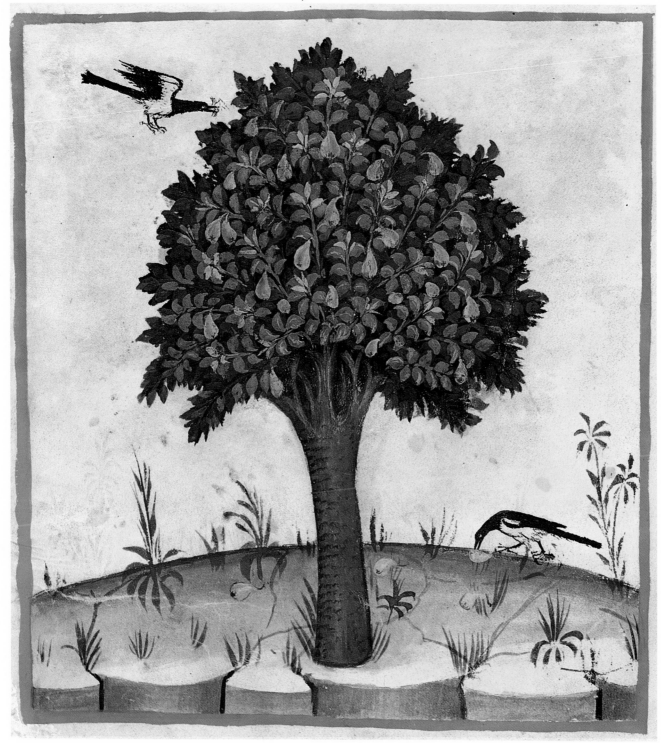

VI

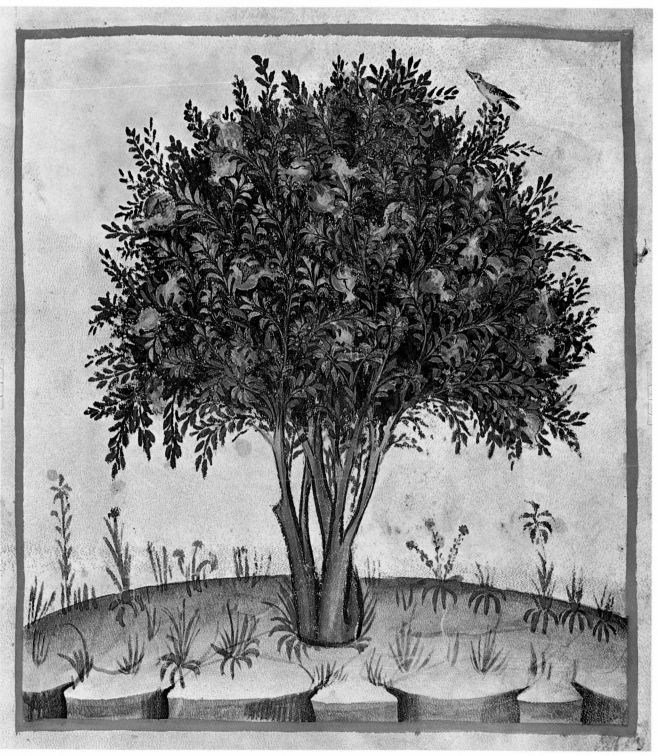

VII

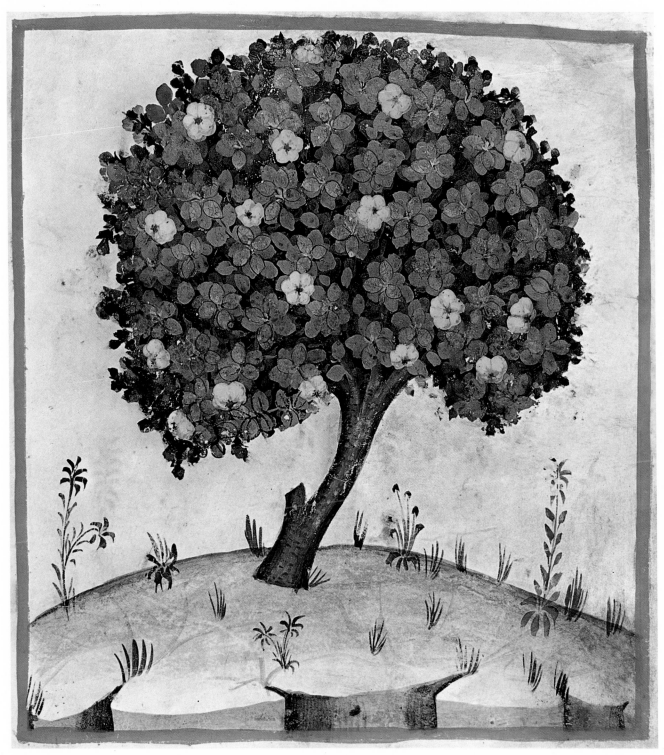

VIII

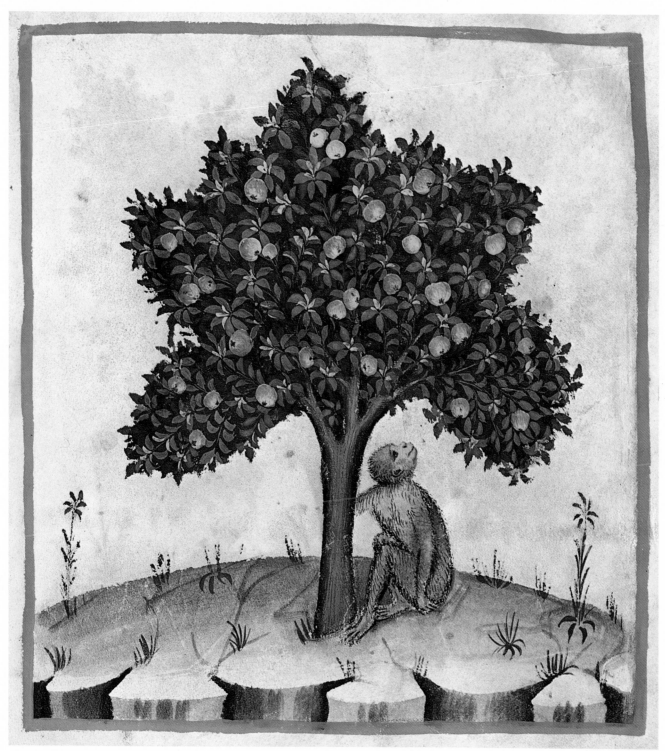

IX

Sicomuri

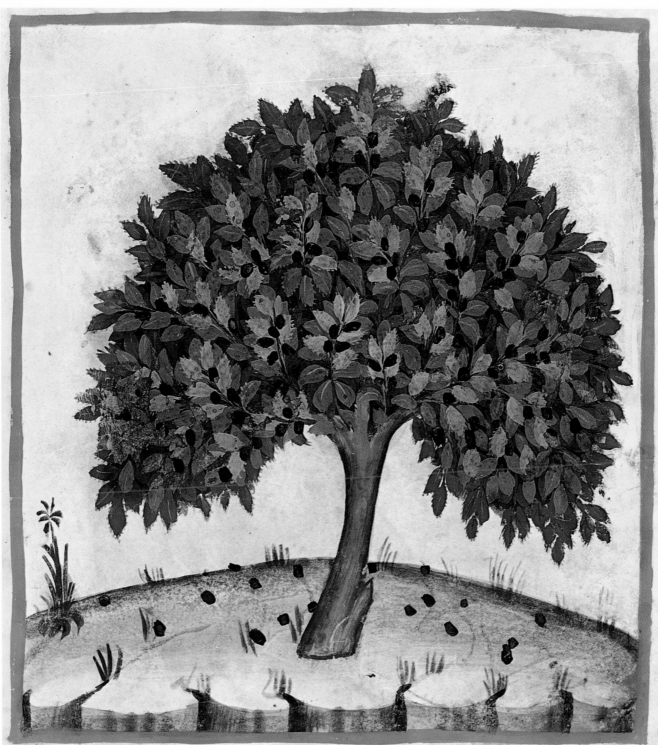

X

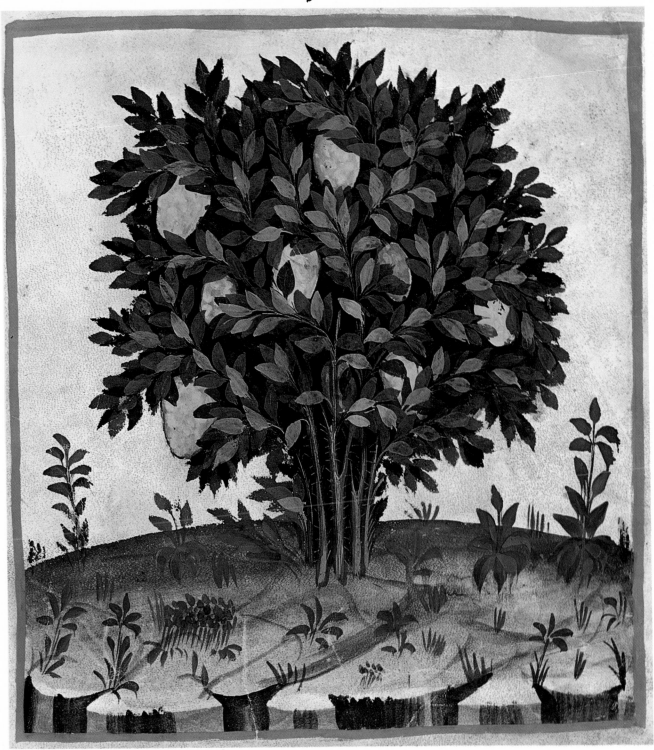

XI

Cerefa dulcia

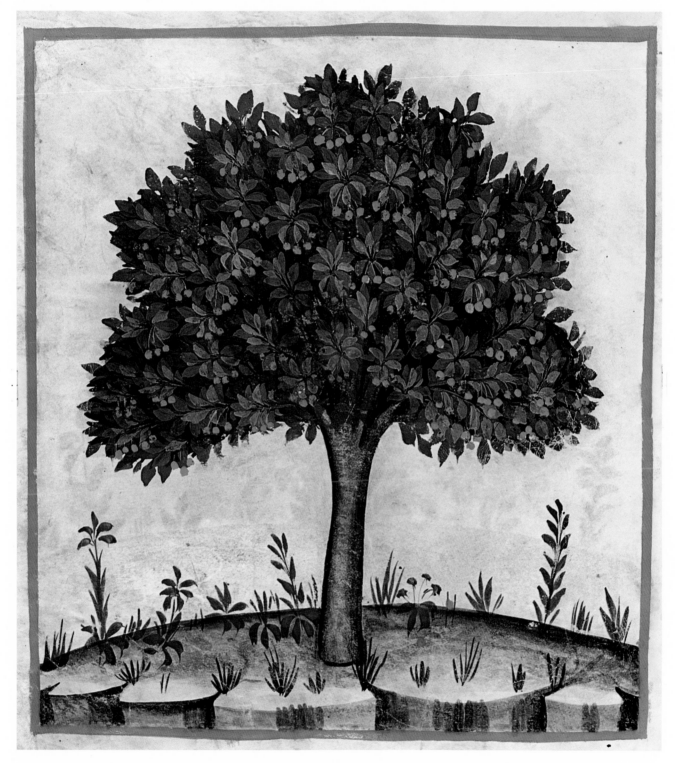

XII

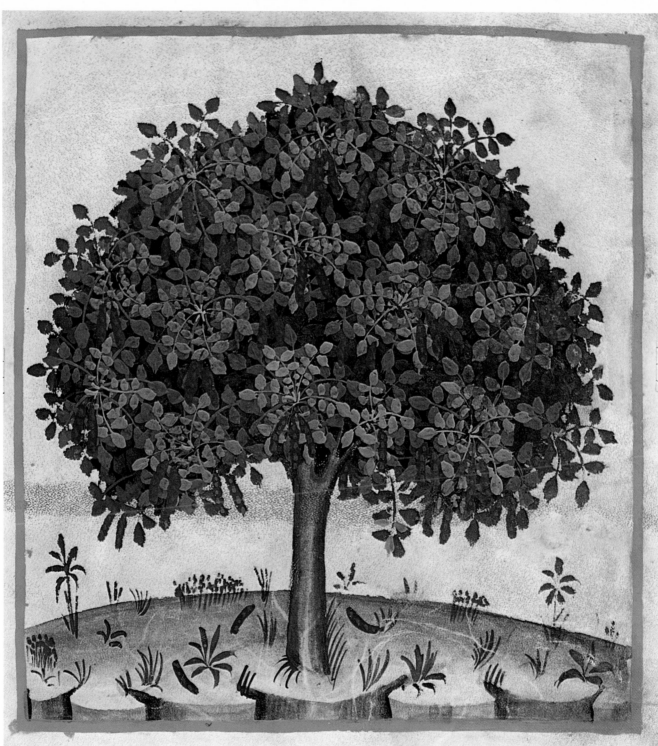

XIII

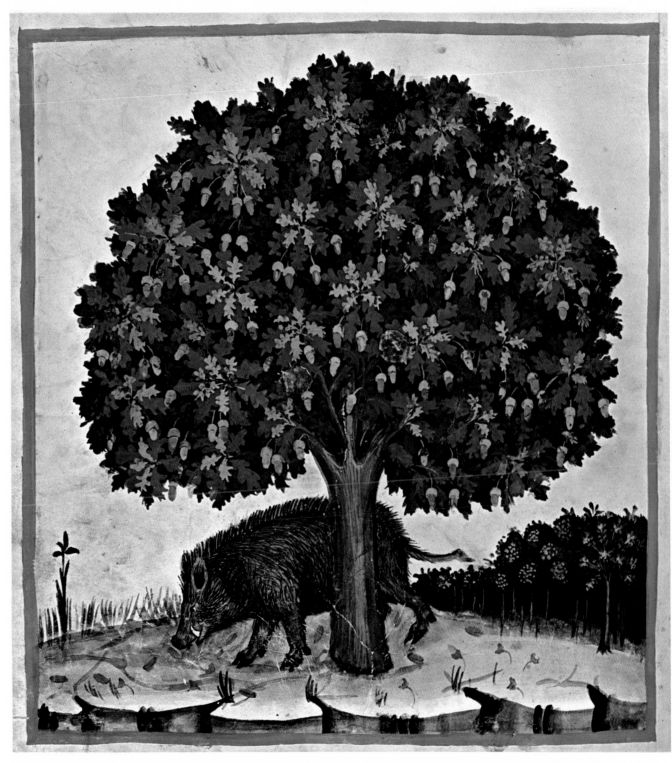

XIV

Oliue nigre.

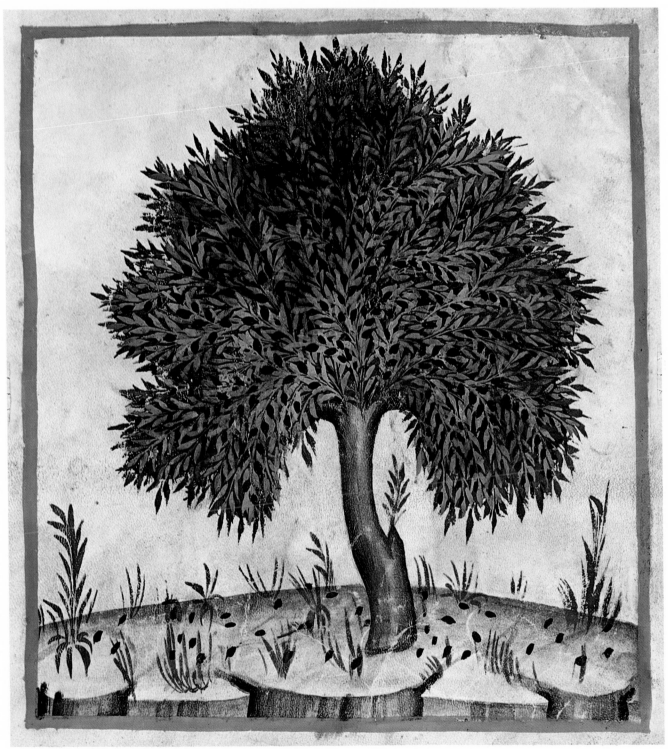

XV

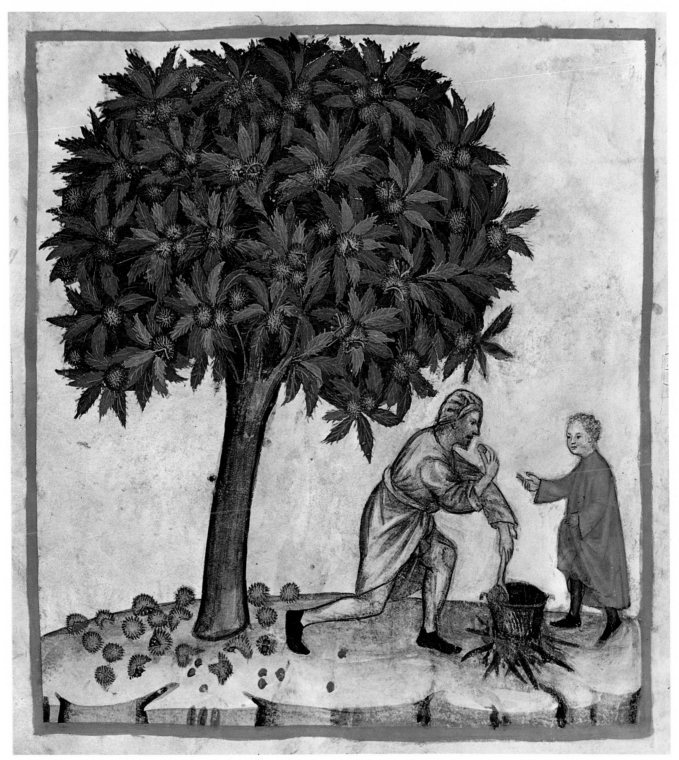

XVI

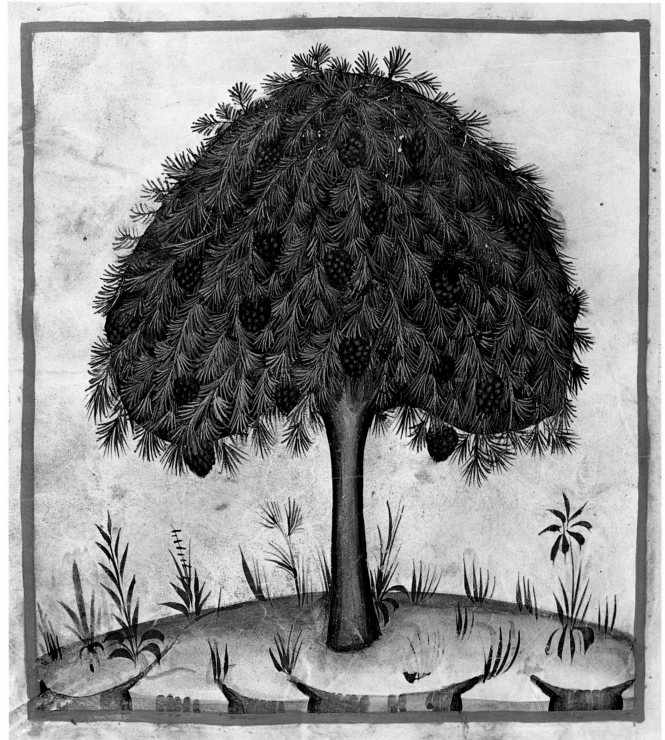

XVII

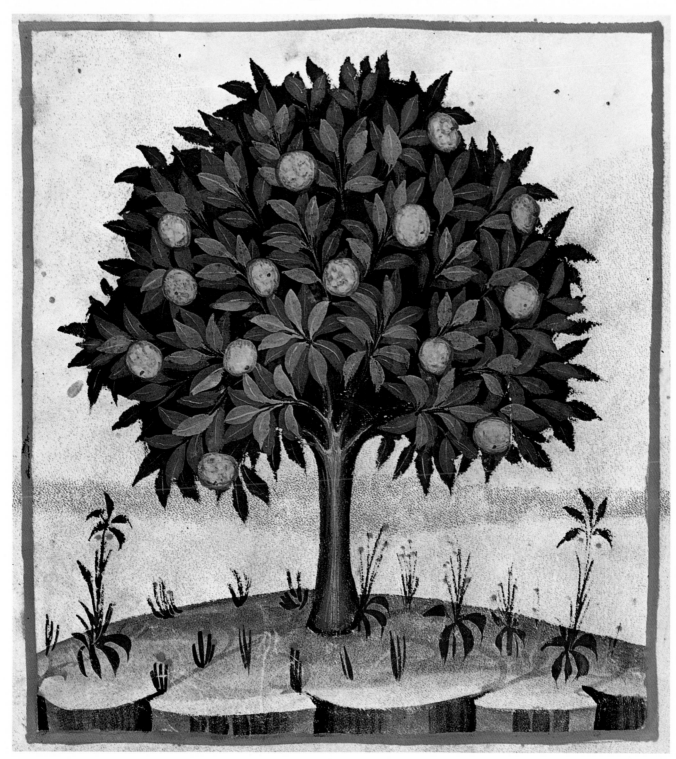

XVIII

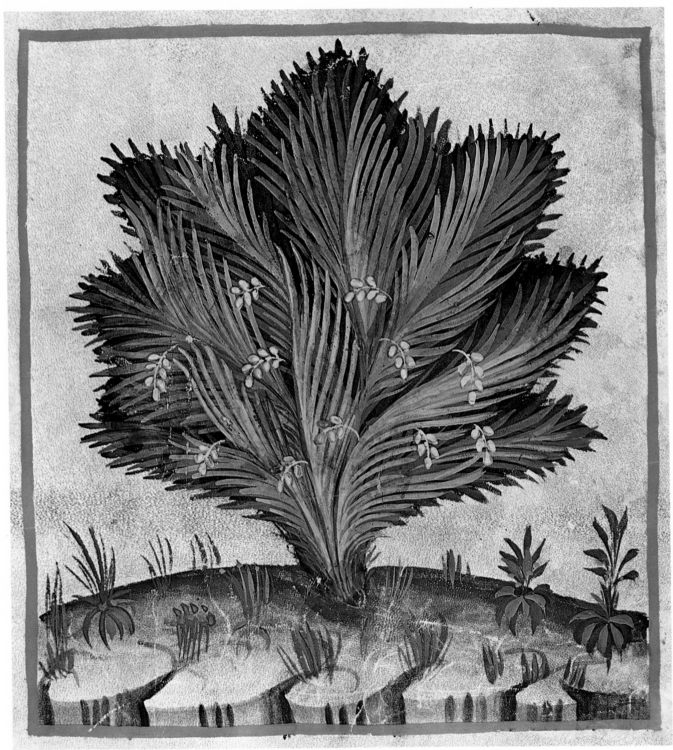

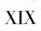

XIX

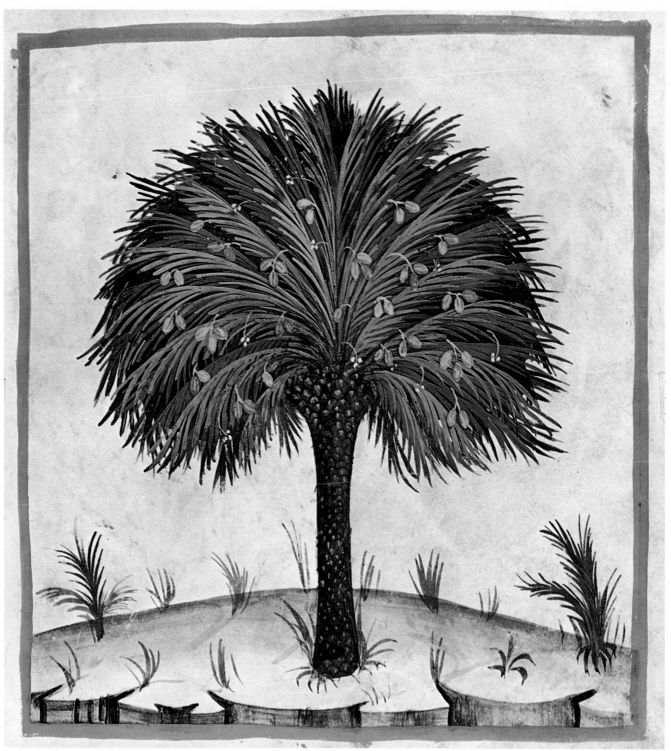

XX

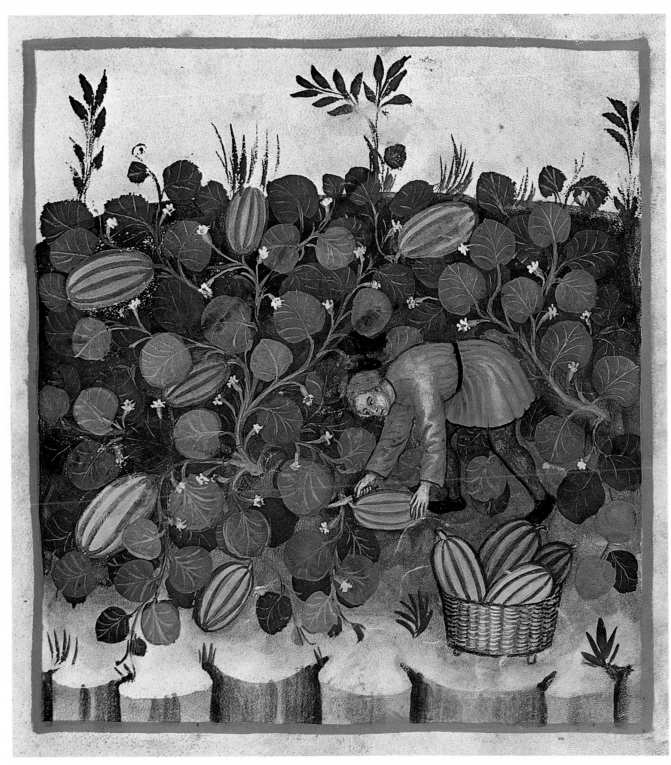

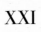

XXI

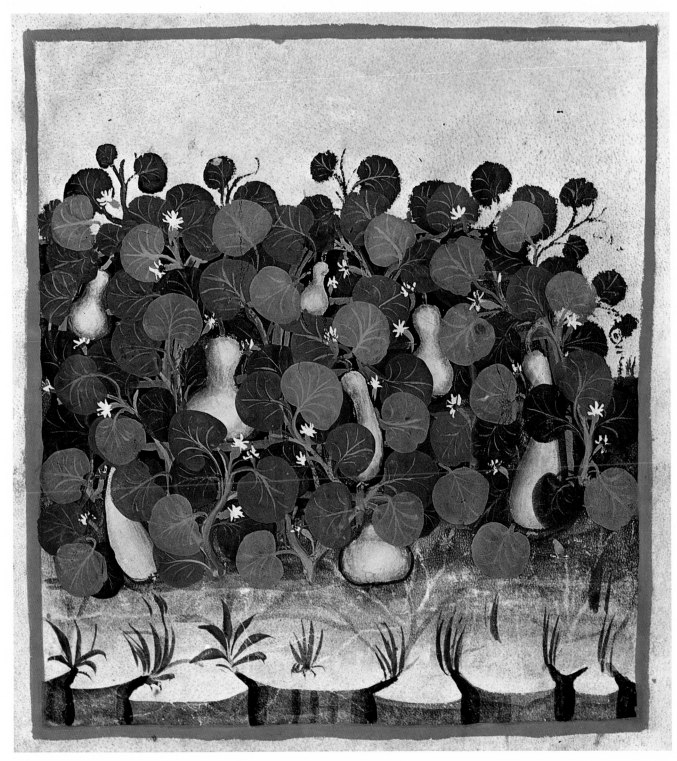

XXII

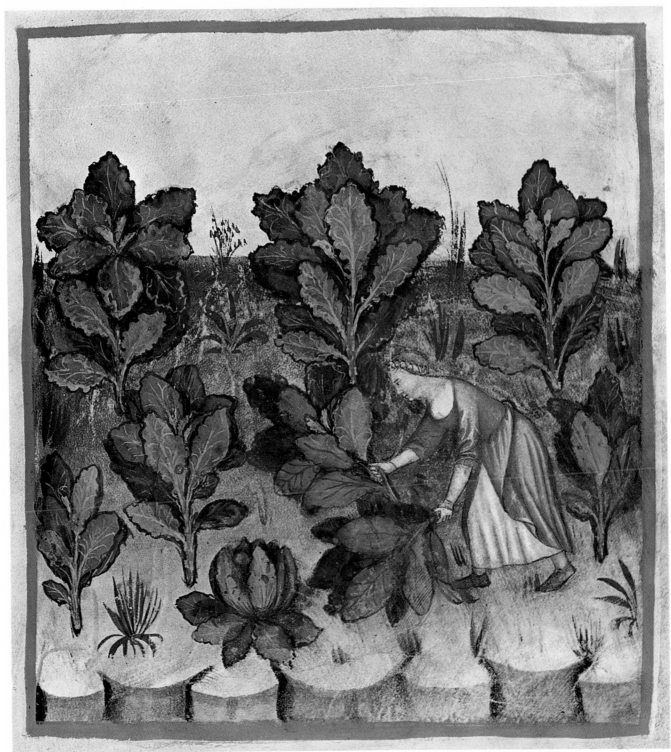

XXIII

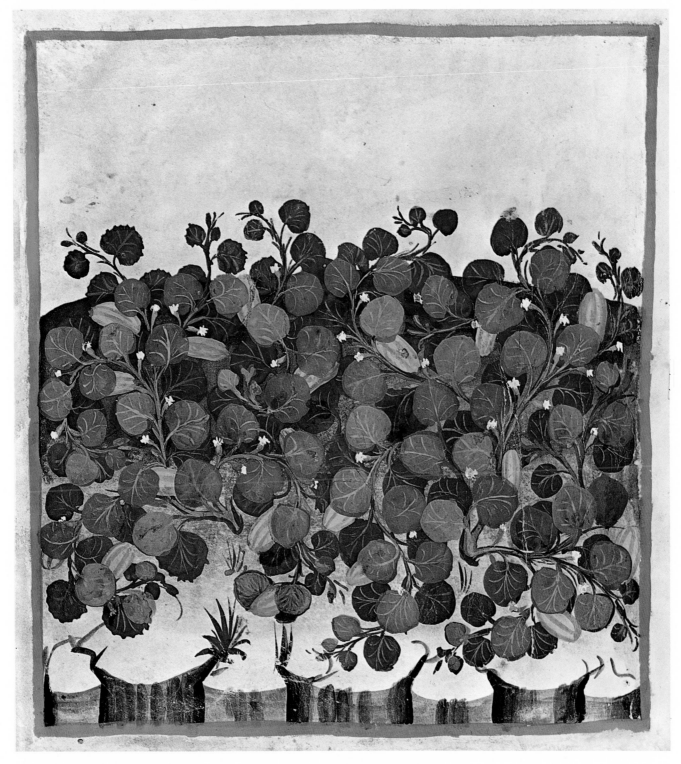

XXIV

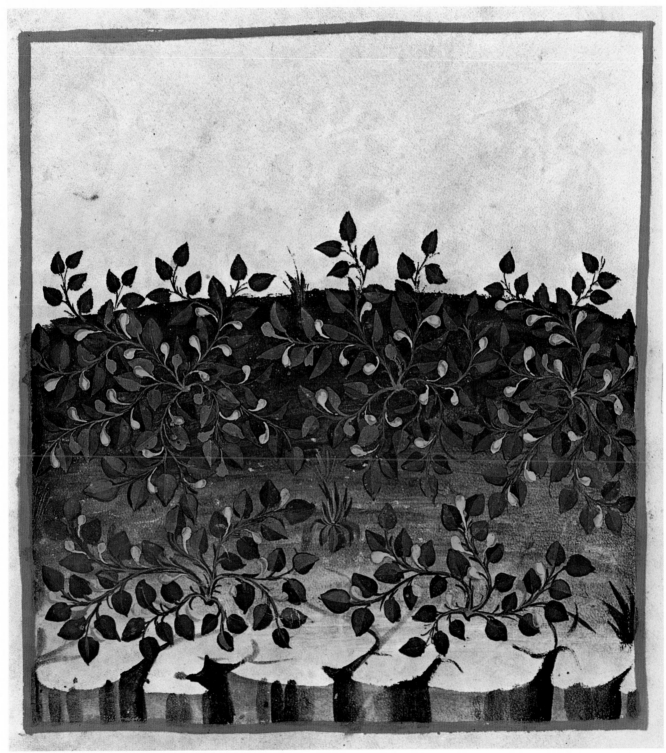

XXV

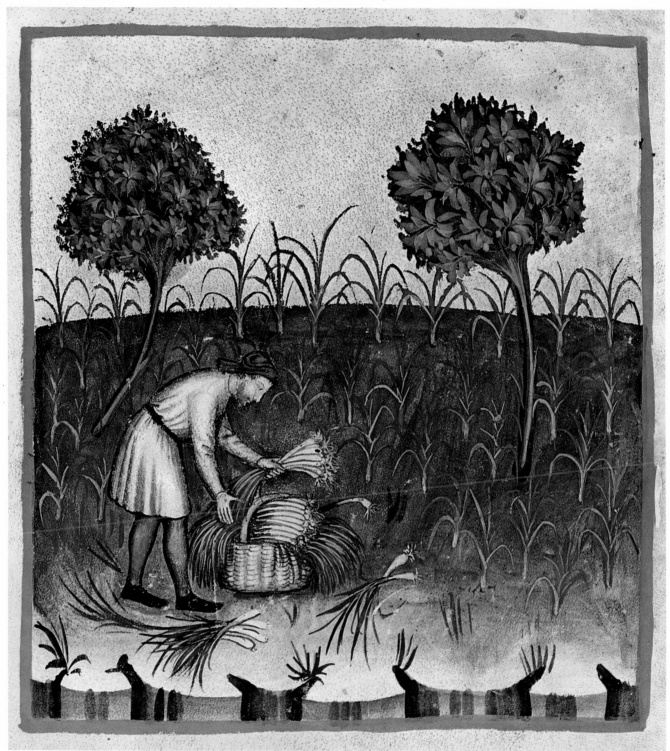

XXVI

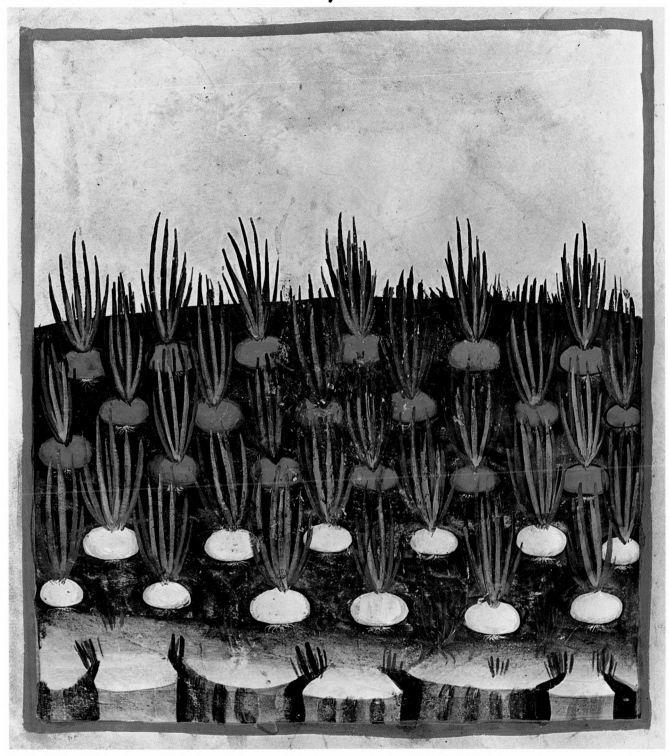

XXVII

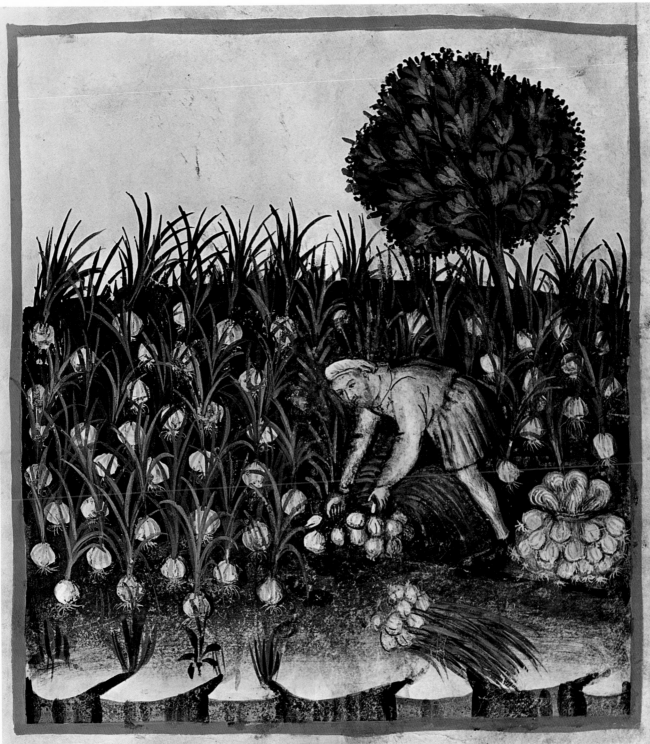

XXVIII

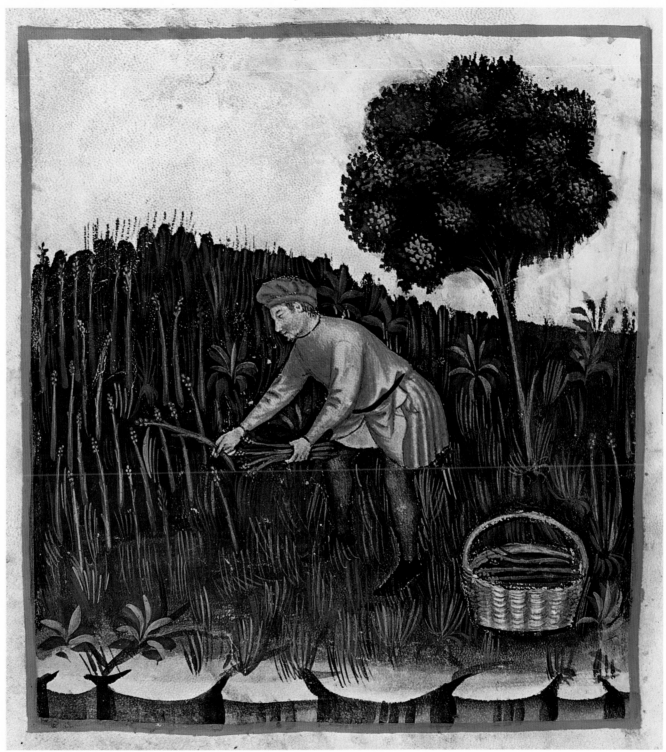

XXIX

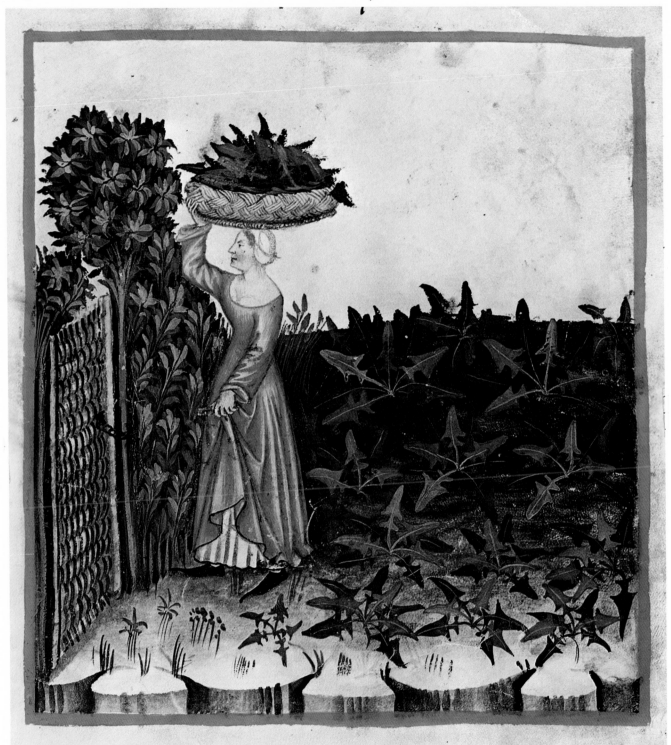

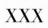

XXX

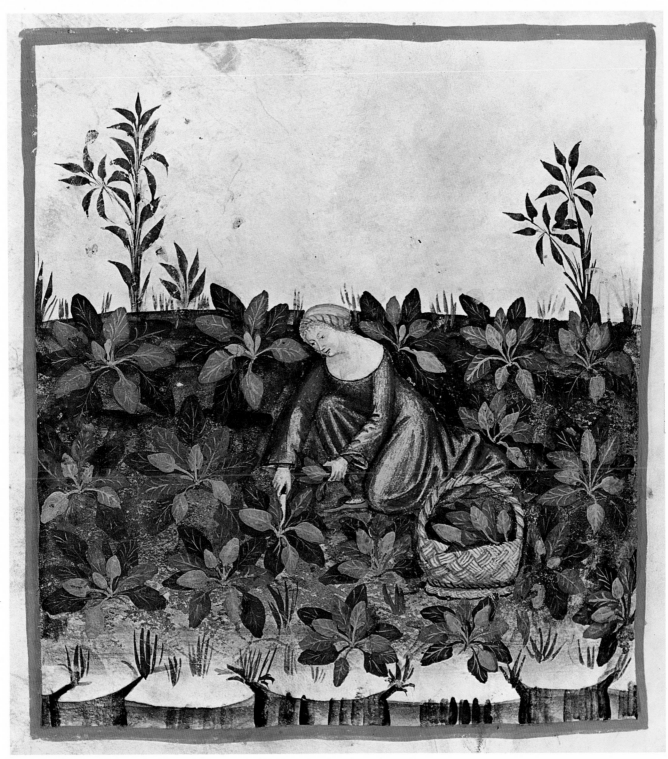

XXXI

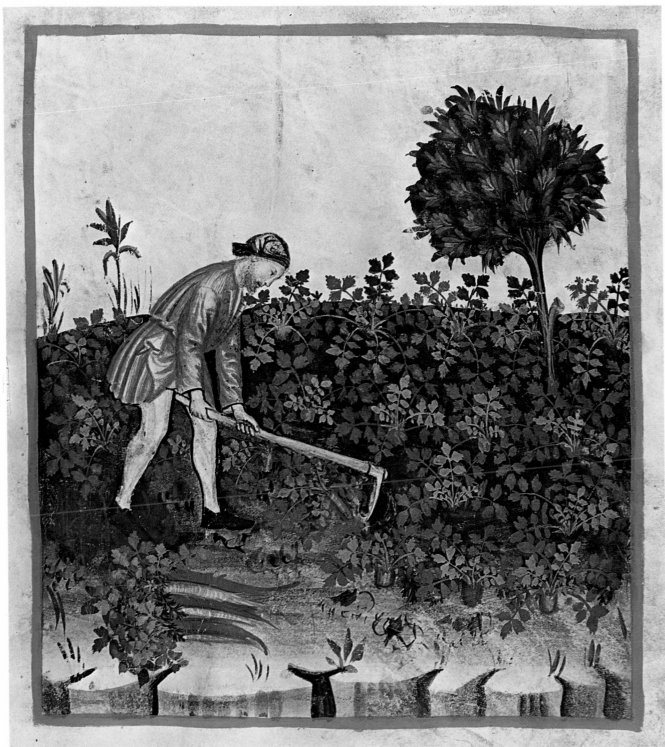

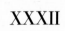
XXXII

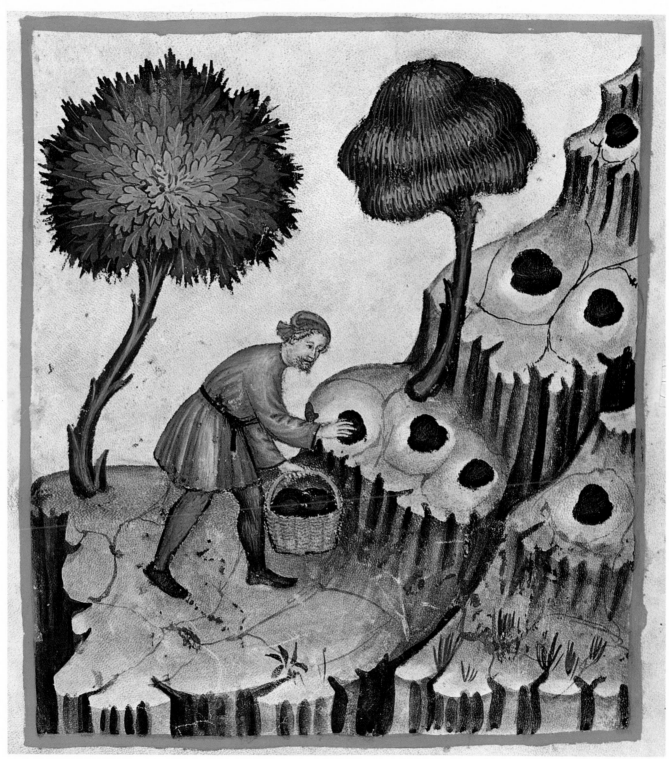

XXXIII

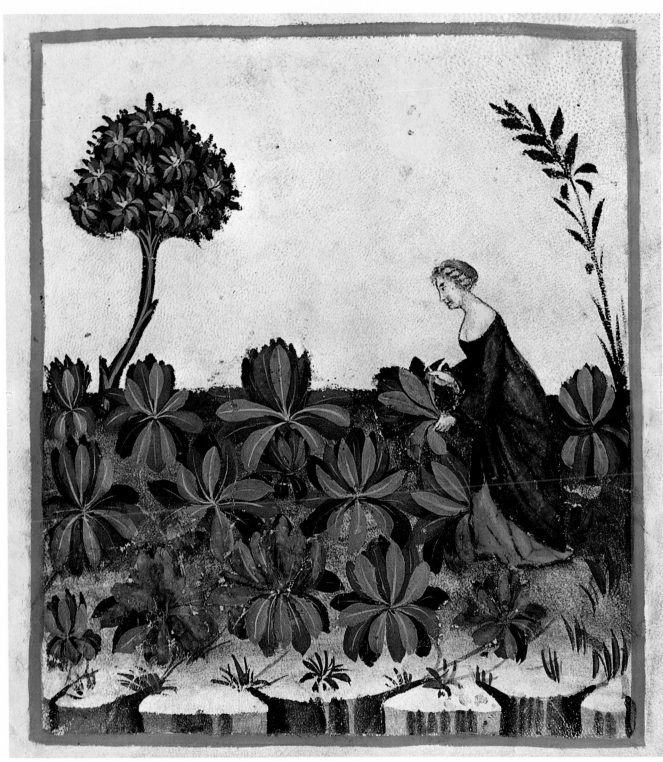

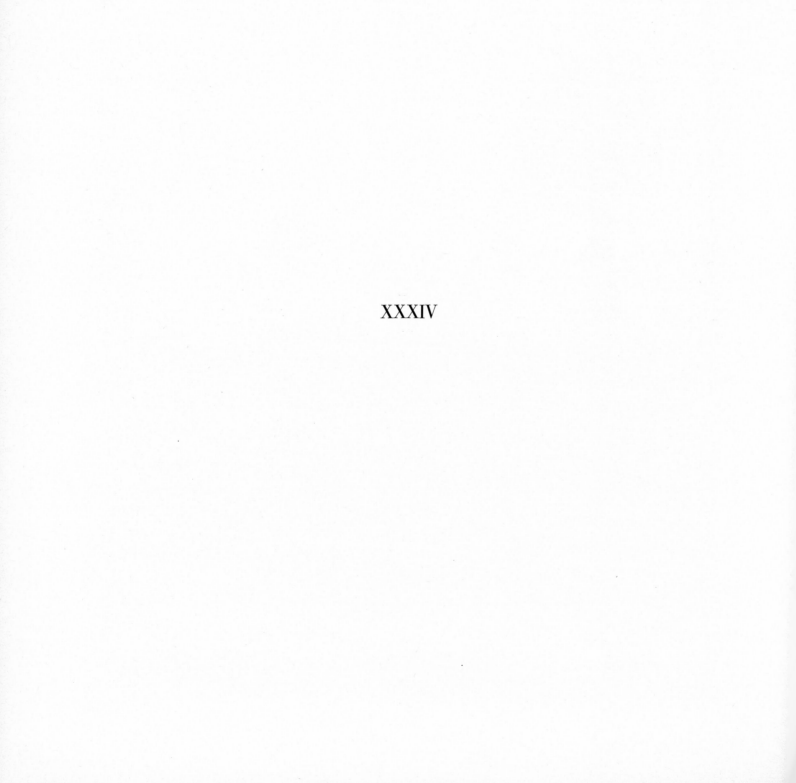

XXXIV

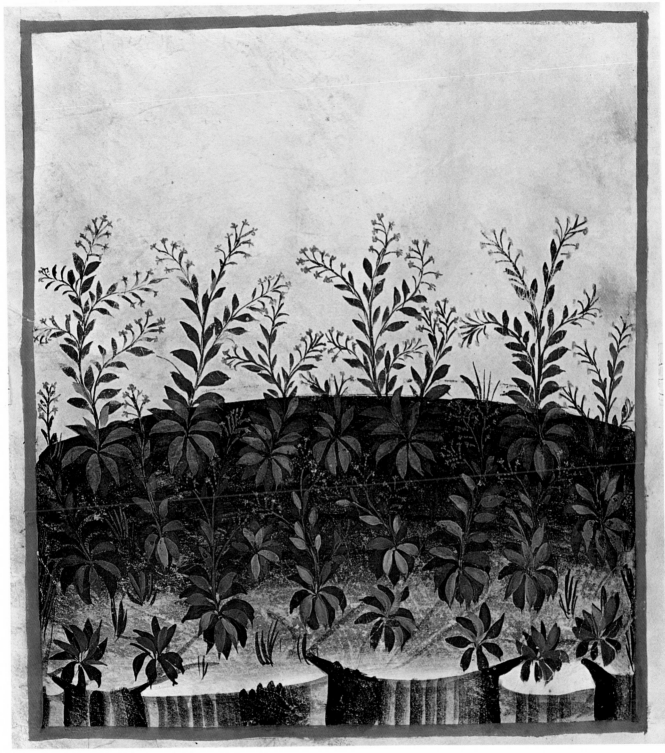

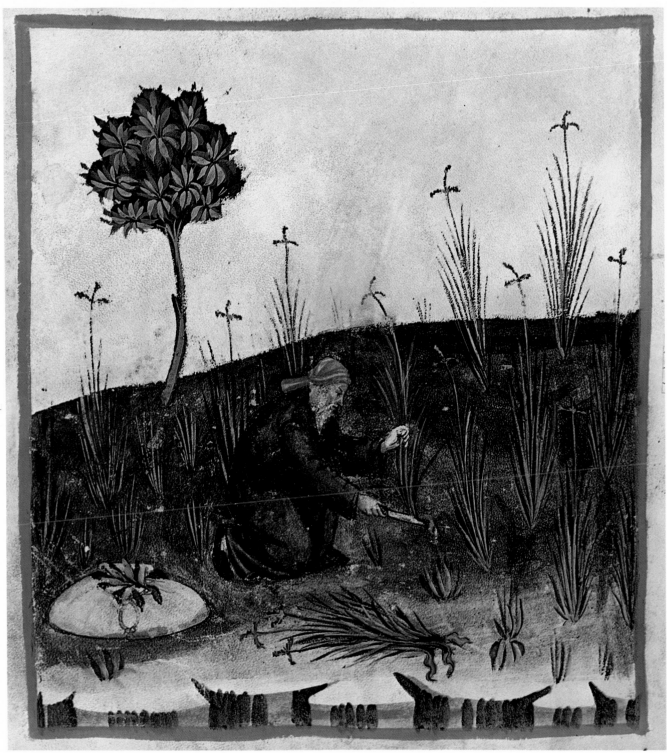

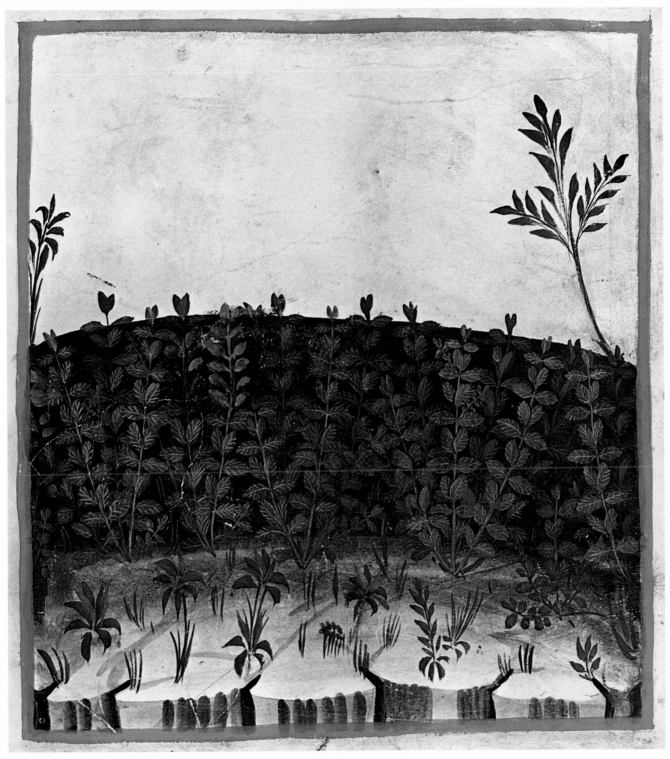

XXXVII

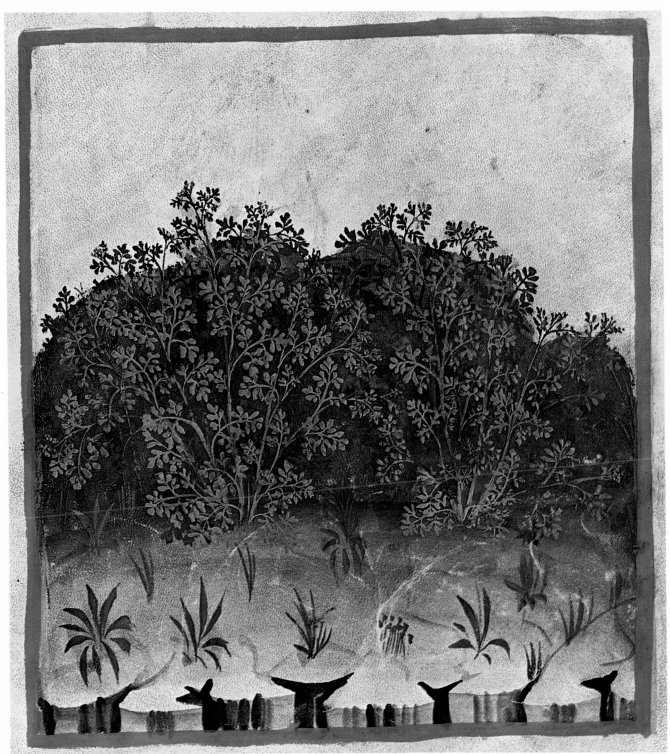

XXXVIII

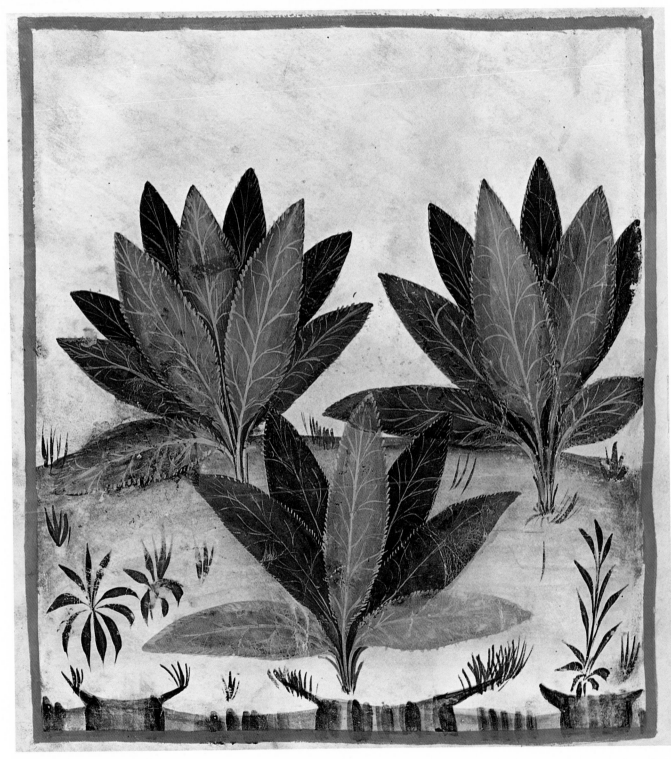

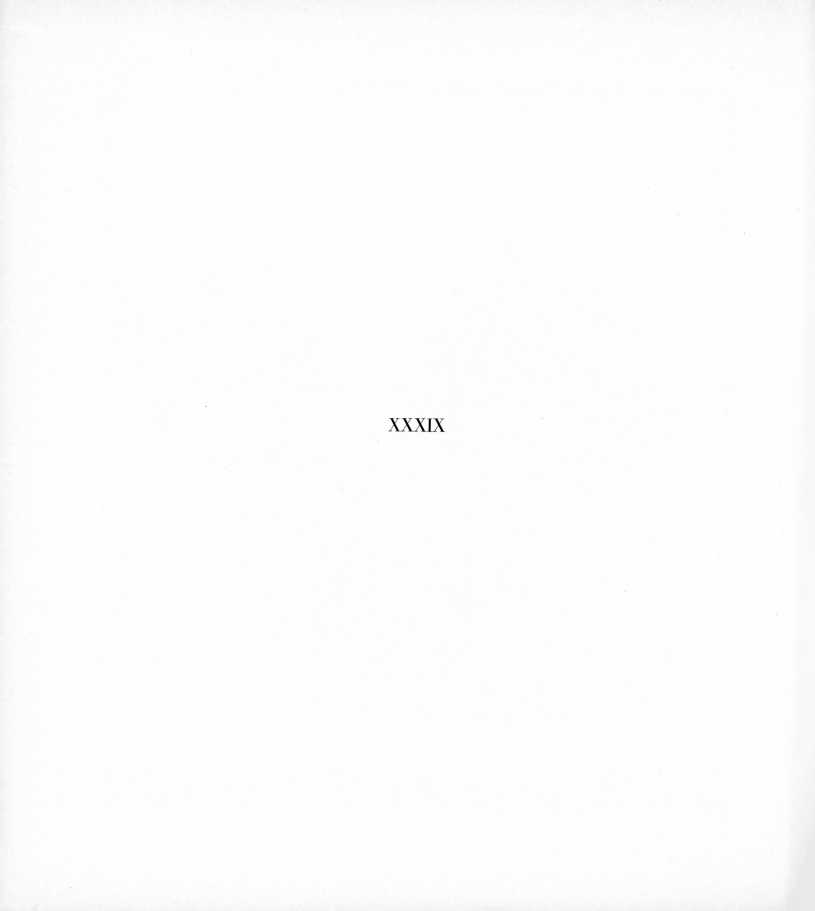

XXXIX

. marubium .

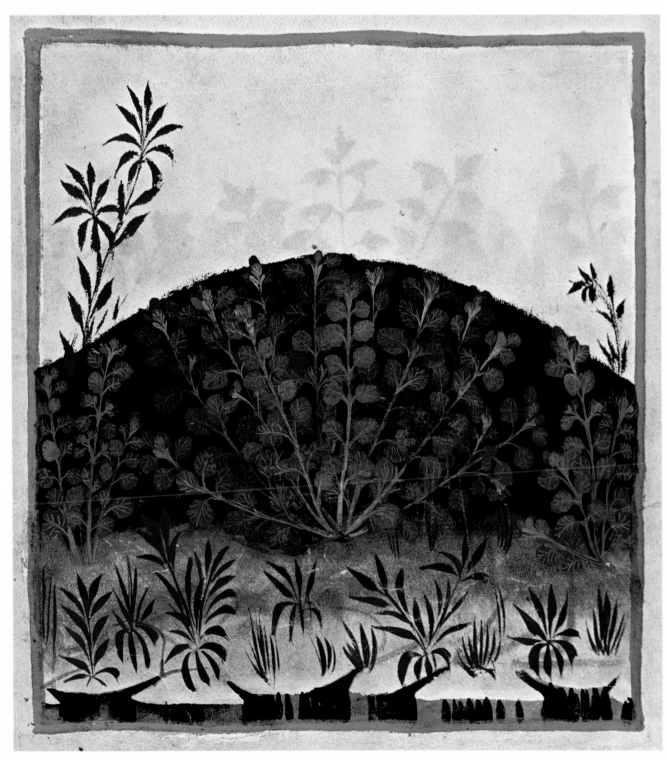

XL

Abſintiũ.

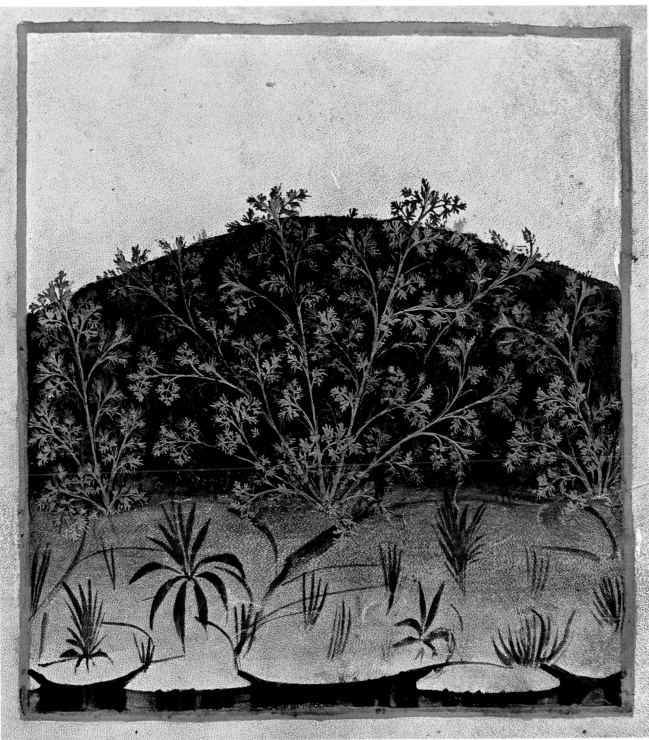

XLI

Saluia

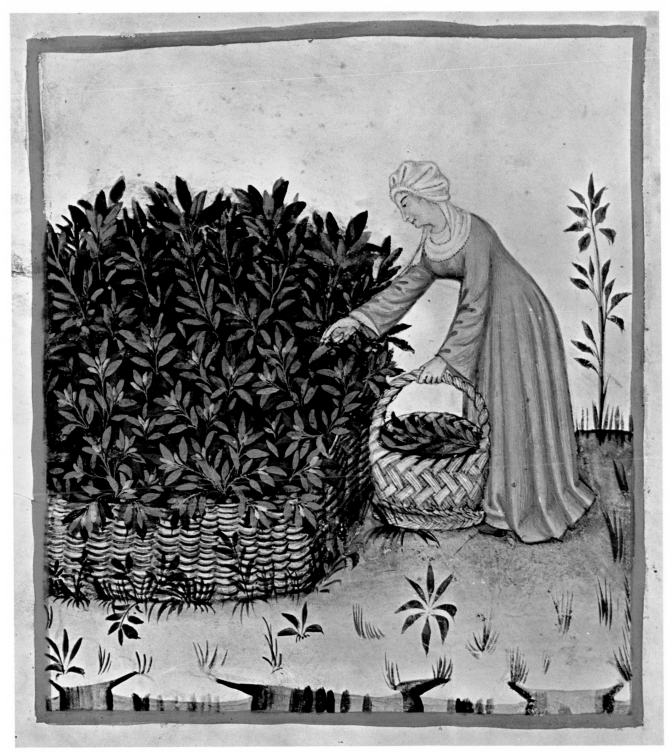

XLII

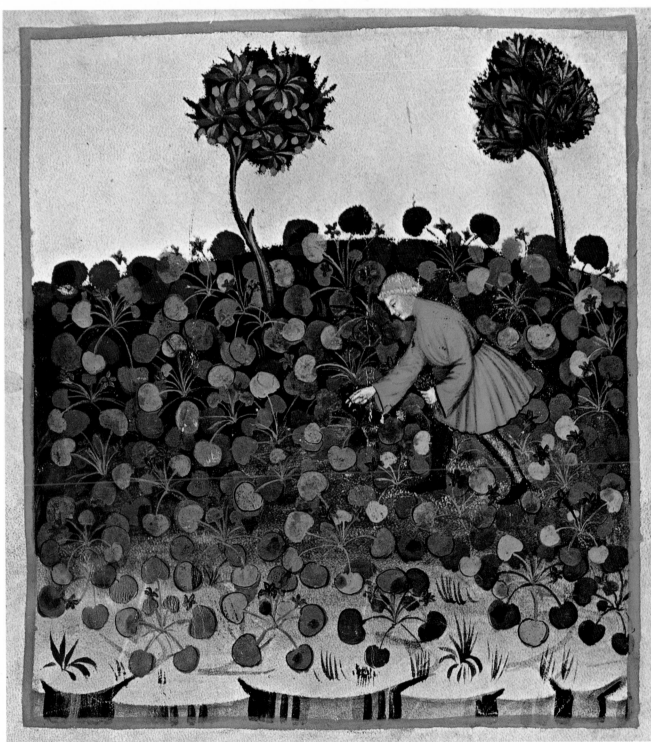

XLIII

Crochus.

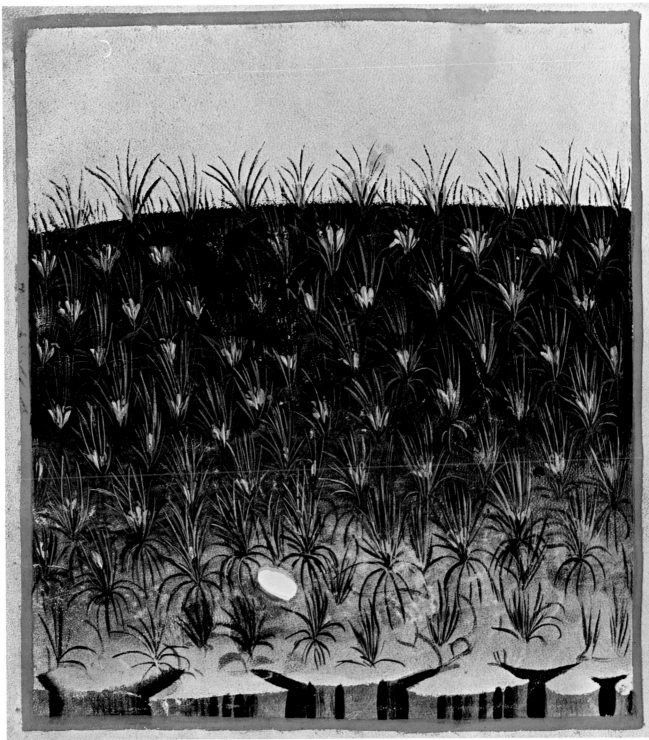

XLIV

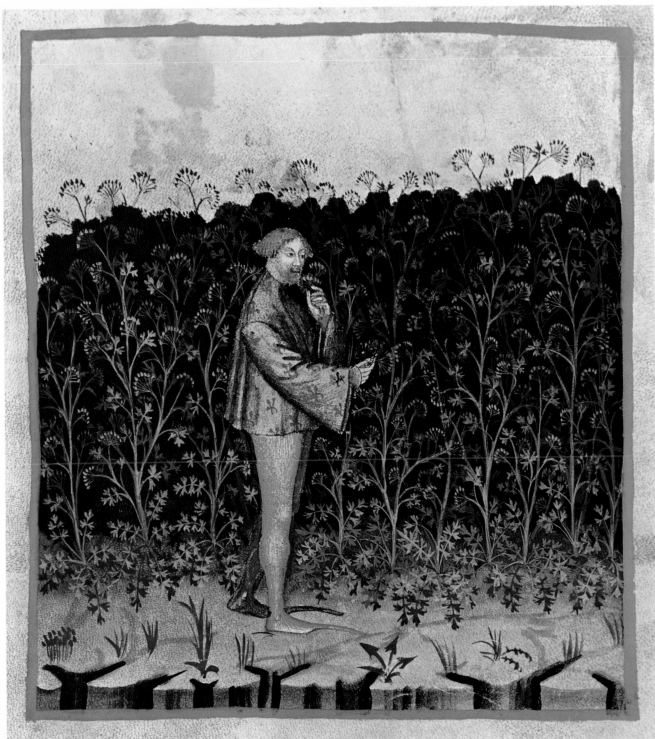

XLV

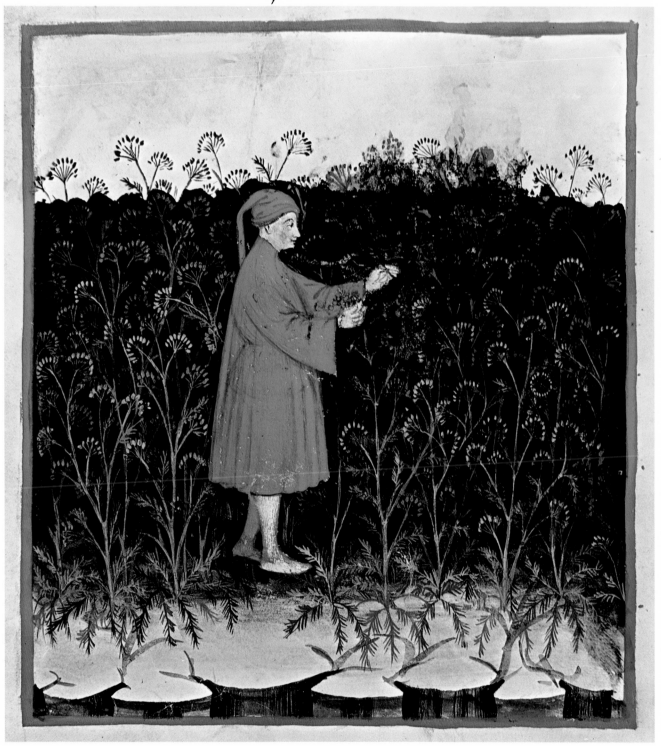

XLVI

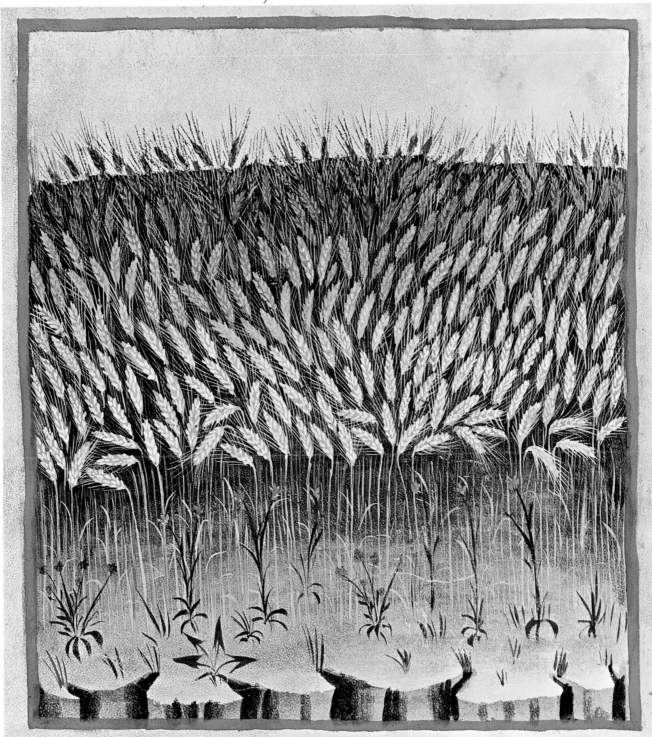

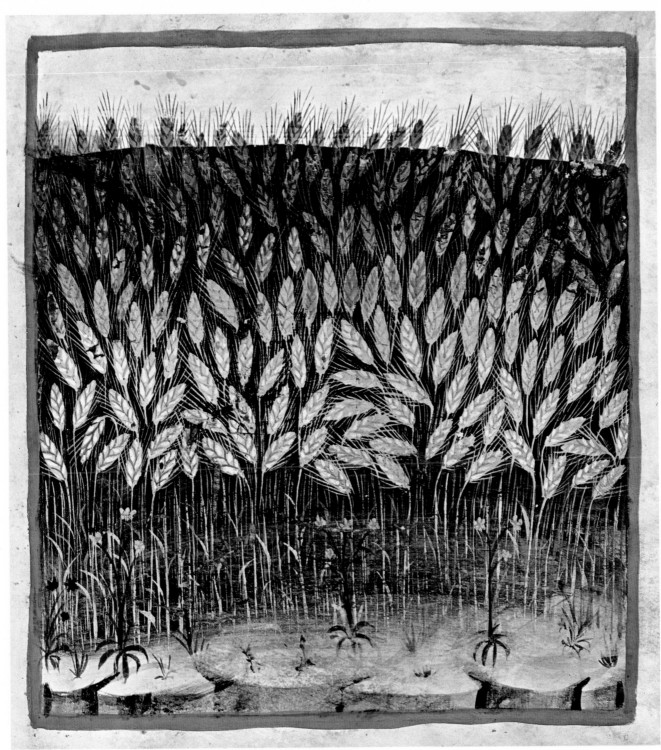